Rock Bottom:

Battle the Addiction From Within

Written By:

James Edward Yorks

Other books include:

Free the Mind: Empowerment Through Improvement

NASCAR Top 100: By A Fan, For the Fans

Bowling Guide 101: Strike Me Now, Spare Me Later

Between The Ropes: Wrestling's Greatest

Contact the Author at:

xtremeneonact@aol.com

203-731-9134

Facebook: James Edward Yorks

Foreword:

When it comes to dealing with addiction, whether it's you or someone you love, we often find ourselves searching for a way up and out. There are countless of ways that addiction destroys our lives. There are numerous types of addictions which we will cover in this book and show that no matter how hard things may be when we're at the lowest of lows, or **Rock Bottom**, we can defeat it from within ourselves. It's not easy, not in a long shot, but it can and will be done. Not everything in this book will deal with just drugs; there are other forms of addiction to cover.

Not by a long shot am I a doctor or someone in the medical field; I am someone who writes this book with experience and someone who has been on both ends of the spectrum when it comes to addiction. I have hit Rock Bottom at one point, I sought for help and everyone kept telling me "you have to want it" and I did. We don't need medical assistance to give one drug to take care of another drug, or habit, we need ourselves. 9 Years coming on 10 of being on top; trust me when I say...follow my lead and you too will find the escape and be able to:

Battle the addiction from within.

Chapters/Index

Chapter 1: What Is Addiction?

Let's start this chapter right out with a given fact that will scare everyone, including you. Everyone at one point in their life has had an addiction, whether they realize it or not. So just know that you or the person that you're trying to help; is *not alone!* How can that be? Let's take a look at what addiction means.

When we look at the scientific statement of addiction, it is when the mind or body needs something so badly that it doesn't seem to work right until it gets its fix. When we look at the dictionary, it states that it's the condition of being addicted to a particular substance, thing, or activity. Medically, same thing however they state that it's something that has to trigger the stimuli in the brain. Addiction starts with a habit and can go out of control which leads us to trouble.

Again, re-read that last paragraph and ask yourself; did I or do I have an addiction? If you can honestly answer that with a firm no, I can strongly suggest that not all addictions are drug related and in the next chapter, I promise you will agree. It sounds harsh, but in reality, we all have had a habit at one time that got away and we became addicted to it.

When we look at someone who suffers with addiction, we often times put blame on them saying that they are bad people or saying that they need "professional or medical help." We have truly become in a state of mind to become quick to judge someone by what they perceive or by the way they look and act. It goes deeper than that; much deeper. When we too can realize that at one point in our life, we can come to understand what is really going on in the mind of someone who has an addiction. Whether it's someone who's addicted to drugs, gambling, shopping, et al. there is hope and a future to help them, or us to be able to get that higher level and out of *Rock Bottom.*

Using the term *Rock Bottom* doesn't fit all of us however. One might say "I've never hit rock bottom" but then doesn't the saying "We have to hit our lowest of lows before we get back on top?"

How does rock bottom and addiction coexist? When we're at rock bottom, we seek help for that quick escape. When we're dealing with addiction, we seek help for that quick escape as well. There are and will forever be ways that we...yes, we can escape and get back on top by doing things our way and from within us.

Let's get into the types of addictions..

Chapter 2: Types of Addiction

This list is just of 28 different topics that we can get into. Under the various; we will talk about the addiction to anti-depressants and uppers/downers, et al. As you can tell, I've pulled some of the drugs out and put them in their own, there's a reason for that. Let's go ahead and get started in this book and hope you're ready to help yourself or a loved one who's currently suffering through addiction.

Alcohol

One of the most powerful addictions; believe it or not that controls our lives comes in the form of alcohol. The substance comes in many ways and for most of us who are in recovery or have had the taste of the drink, it's not easy to give up; nor is it hard to resist. In fact, many of us who have walked away are tempted daily especially with knowing how it cured our problems temporarily.

Sure, there are some out there who say it's only one drink, it won't hurt; how many people do we know that have only had 1 drink and been able to never sip it again? Ever been to a fancy restaurant where they offer "Beer battered shrimp?" Alcohol burns off when cooking, but it's still in the mind when you're dealing with the disease and addiction of alcoholism that you can have a glass of water and think you're drinking vodka.

The problem with alcohol is not only it's long term effects on what it does to the body, but also what it does mentally, physically and emotionally. It can also destroy lives by turning family members; or costing you the job that you're working to supply the *habit*. I'm using the term habit very loosely here.

Consuming alcohol is not a habit, nor can anyone tell me that they can do it socially and live a comfortable life. When we have a bottle of wine for holidays or have to have that drink to celebrate an event, it turns to a yearly event. Can you do it with soda, water, juice? Sure. But there's always one person in every crowd that has to say "pop the champagne because it's not right." Agree with me or not on this part, but if you have to have the drink (even if it's once a year) you are addicted.

Now it won't destroy your life, but if you have more than that one, you are now over the legal limit to drive. Get behind the wheel and now you're not only risking your life, but the lives of others. Get behind the wheel and you might have a date with the local or state law enforcement. Is it worth the risk?

Being a social drinker can also affect your life by messing up your schedule. When at the bar with friends on a night out, one friend leaves and now another straggles in. Next thing you know; you planned on leaving at 7pm and it's not 10 or 11. If you have to be up at 5:30 to walk the dog and head to work, you now didn't get the full night of sleep which now can affect your commute or even performance of the job. Do this enough times and your boss notices...bye job.

Say you have a great family and you fully support them. If you're spending all your hard earned money at the bar, it can lead to a bad ending. Too many families are being broken up due to alcohol. There are some who just drives them into a deeper rut because they can't handle with how it got so messed up. Now sadly, you and the pet are living in the car or having to move around because you lost that big house, fancy car, and pretty family. All because alcohol came in.

These are just three scenarios of the countless amounts of ways that alcohol can and will destroy lives. Out of the thousands of people that I've already come across in my travels from a previous book; Free the Mind: Empowerment Through Improvement; I've seen it and heard it all too often. Through the people that I come across at social gatherings and in the "rooms" I've heard war stories. It all comes down to the same ending.

So how can we fix ourselves to end the problem? What if we really are addicted to the taste or scent of alcohol? How did we get so out of touch and lose control that badly? Is there a way for us to really put down that drink and never walk back to it? Why so many questions when there's really one simple answer.

When it comes to fixing the problem and getting alcohol out of our lives, the battle really does start from within. We can turn it down but then peer pressure sets in and we're worried about what our friends or family think of us; especially if it's "uncle randy" over there in the corner saying...it's only 1.

I'm not going to stand here and lie by saying that the scent and taste of alcohol isn't intriguing. I will say that when walking in a bar and seeing the drunk guy in the corner is not who I want to end up being by the end of the night; nor should you.

Walking away from alcohol is always hard regardless of how much time you have invested, or when we say "I'll never do that again." So how do we find the inner strength to win the battle? Believe it or not, there's a couple ways.

First; get a different beverage. It can be anything really; sodas, water, juice, punch. Some places might even let you bring your own. Second; explore a different route. If it's in the routine on the way home, go a different way home. Third; if you knew anyone who died from alcoholism or any of the cancers that go with it, carry their picture in your wallet. If you can't beat it on your own, then yes, there are the rooms of Alcoholics Anonymous.

Amphetamine

Often times, this drug is not a lethal drug, but it is a highly addictive drug due to the effects one can get from usage. When it becomes dangerous is when it's mixed with other habitual usages like alcohol. It does affect the Central Nervous System and can still be dangerous due to it being a stimulant. When doctors give us this drug, they don't use it by name; and most people don't know that they are taking it. Some of the most common street names are as follows; Adderall, Dexedrine, Meth, Ritalin, and Levoamphetamine.

College kids struggle with this especially when it comes time to do exams and they are doing the cram sessions. If you are a parent and ever hear your child talking about some of these names, the awareness should be raised; Bennies, Molly, Jelly Beans, Oranges, and Fast Lightning. Again, mixed with alcohol, it can lead to death. With alcohol causing your heart and brain to go slower, and amphetamines causing your heart to go faster, it can lead to heart failure and brain damage.

To win the battle against this drug is really not to get involved with it in the first place, unless under doctors care. If you've already started it, take a time out and count to 20. You can also learn meditation.

Analgesics

One of the most common drugs that become highly addictive under a different name without knowledge is Analgesics; better known as painkillers. Just this one topic alone could cover pretty much any and all types of drugs. When we use drugs, we seek to find an escape, or relief, from whatever it is that's ailing us. It doesn't matter if it's a long term escape or short term; *everything* has its addictions and troubles that will have permanent effects.

Painkillers are especially dangerous because when taking them for an ailment and the pain doesn't subside, the user wants to take more thinking that it will change, and can lead to an overdose. There is no easy way to describe the amount of pain that they actually cause. There is no easy way to describe how they can and will destroy life as you know it. Though most of the drugs are prescribed by doctors, there are other escapes that can be purchased over the counter and can be highly addictive as well.

Painkillers can be as little as aspirin, Tylenol, alcohol, opioids, marijuana or as high as drugs prescribed by doctors. Painkillers come in many ways shapes and form. How do we know if we're addicted to them and what can we do to get away from them?

If it's from dealing with a cold or headache, then that's one thing. But some of us, who have that addictive personality, can't take it just for the sake of getting rid of a headache. Two pills then turn into 4 for body aches which turns into searching for more or a stronger drug to heal the pain. When we chase that feeling of relief, or the betterment to escape our pain, it all leads to the same dark road.

Believe it or not, we all chased that dark road at one point of our life. We've all been addicted to a painkiller at one point. Perhaps we still are just without knowledge. Every time we feel an ache or pain, we just naturally reach for that bottle of aspirin, or ibuprofen to get the pain to go away. We have a cough, we take cough medicine. We do what we're told to do because we don't like the feeling and don't want it to get worse, but in essence, we are naturally setting ourselves up for an addiction that will last a lifetime.

There is no real way to break the addiction from painkillers just because we have been trained from such a young age. We can try to block out the pain and do classic meditation, go for a walk, communicate with others about our ailment. We can do soup for sore throat as we already do, and seek other ways to self-medicate, but we have to know our limits on dosage.

Appearance

It's safe to say that society has led us to this addiction. How is our appearance an addiction? Ever hear of the term "dress to impress?" This goes for all genders. We are constantly worried about how we dress or how we act because that's the way society has affected us from a very young age.

Do you remember the time when it was okay to just wear sweats or pajamas out in public and not have to worry about being frowned upon? Believe it or not, this was the case up until 2008. Some of us still have that no frills, take me as I am attitude, but in hindsight, we are still looked down upon. How can it be? We are called lazy because we don't want to get dressed if it's only a morning run for a cup of coffee; We are called grungy if we don't comb our hair if only running to the store; we are called dirty if we don't take a quick morning shower before leaving the house..even on our day off from work when it's our relaxation day.

Society has set us up to be more concerned about our looks and appearance to the public more than ever; this is the same society who shouts for anti-bullying. Are we all not guilty of looking at someone and saying something along the lines of "can't they afford new sneakers or jeans without holes in them?"

This can lead to a long road of loneliness, not just as the victim but as the tormentor. We all are capable of having the addiction to satisfying others needs before ourselves.

We can defeat society and we can beat this addiction both in one shot. It's the starting of a new chapter in our lives, and we can change this addiction by being different. How is this possible? Take the challenge and one day, don't be afraid to go out in sweats or pajamas and do a neighborhood store run or do your errands and if anyone says anything, just comment that it's a new look. Sounds hard, but don't we go to a paper box, or mailbox, or walk our family pet and not care what anyone says or what they do? Why should it be different any other time?

To beat this addiction from within, it's the easiest and possibly the most fun way possible. It can also lead to the start of a new beginning that can also change other things in life. There should be one day, like we used to have back in school, where it's okay for everyone to wear pajamas out in public; sadly we have aged and it's frowned upon to be different. I say it's time to go back to it and have fun. Find funny pair if possible, let people know that it's your day, and make them want to be...just...like...you!

Benzo's

Benzodiapamine, better known as Benzo's are a psychedelic drug that was actually discovered by accident. It reached its high point of usage in the world in the 70's and has remained on the scene through the test of time. They are popular with kids these days as an experimental drug and need to be dealt with as they are being combined with other drugs and lead to an all-time high in fatalities by overdoses.

Some of the reasons why Benzo's are still actively used to this day and why they are part of an addiction that are due to what they are used for and how they are prescribed. They are prescribed for dealing with alcohol dependence, panic attacks, anxiety disorders, and insomnia. Under hospital care, they are given through an IV; through recreational use, they are done with needles or even rectally.

The problem with Benzo's is that they can induce a level of comfort that someone feels at peace with and can become highly addicted to it. As someone who has had a problem with addiction in the past or even currently, it is still a drug that can end a life due to the long term effects. Most doctors try to prescribe it for short term, but as an addict enjoys the feeling, they tend to mix with other drugs and get hooked longer.

Some can say that they aren't dangerous; already had a couple of arguments with people in the medical field as I mentioned about writing this book. But let's just say that the person who's using Benzo's to cure anxiety. Now they run out and have a few beers with friends. First and foremost, being a psychedelic drug, they don't belong out on the road in the first place; now you add alcohol to the mix. Same thing as we mentioned before, it is a deadly combination.

Why would doctors give us something that can lead to death? Can it be placed in the wrong hands? Of course and the problem is that as we have problems dealing with addiction, regardless of what type of addiction, we sometimes don't consider ourselves an addict and not all doctors ask about "drug of choice."

To get away from Benzo's is to first educate yourself on what you're putting in your body. Is it harmful and cause long-term effects? As we can say that with everything that we come in contact with throughout our lives, this is one drug that regardless of the situation, we need to make sure this does not come in contact within. It can and will do long-term damage and we need to keep this away from our kids. Too many are dying from experimenting with this.

Caffeine

The infamous drug that we all are addicted to without a shadow of a doubt; caffeine. Though it's a legal drug, caffeine is something that is a product of addiction. Whether it's in our coffee, tea, soda, beans, products we eat, or straight up injecting it (yes, there are some people out there who do that) it's a daily part of our lives.

For the coffee lovers out there, not saying anyone will or has tried this; it takes a 82 cups of coffee in one sitting for a 180 pound man to die of an overdose of caffeine. On a personal note, I drink around 15 cups of a coffee a day (which equates to 3 pots a day) and I can tell you that I am on the run afterwards. Add nicotine to the mix, and your heart is on the run out of the chest and there's no hope; been there, done that.

Back to the serious side of caffeine though, it does come in many shapes and forms. There are ways that we can say we drink decaf or aim for caffeine-free products, but unless we read the labels and know the other names of the product, there is still a touch of caffeine or other additives in it. Caffeine is a stimulant that can have numerous side effects that can affect your daily routine and hurt in the same sense.

As with coffee, caffeine is in our daily intake especially if we are soda drinkers. I can't reiterate enough that even though its caffeine free, there are other stuff that's in the beverage that's just as dangerous if not worse. Most of the soda companies tried at one time to remove aspartame, which is an artificial sweetener.

If you, as some people do, believe everything that you read on the internet (it's there, it must be true right?) then there was a rumor back in the day. It was linked to lupus, cancer, spasms, blindness and more. They have all been proven to be false which led to adding it back into soft drinks.

Caffeine is found in all soft drinks, not just cola. In fact, some of your better known sodas have more caffeine in them than cola can begin to shake a stick at. Products like Root Beer contain a 2:1 ratio in it so next time you have that Root Beer Float with that delicious Vanilla Ice Cream, think about it. Then there's cream soda, grape soda, and all the other types of soda. Not only the caffeine but other chemicals that can do bodily harm and rot teeth, as well as the fats and sugars that can and will destroy your body from within.

Sticking with caffeine, and off to the lighter side, there's something else we need to discuss. Something that's just as detrimental to our health when taking it.

There are also some of us out there who have taken caffeine pills for the morning uppers while waiting for the coffee to kick in. This is just plain dangerous without knowing it. Granted, we might feel the need for it but it's highly addictive. Those who are in young ages and taking them for study sessions or looking for that quick jolt. Kids these days are popping one after another and then mixing them with alcohol which is severely dangerous to the heart as well as other organs. Also have people crushing them up and snorting them; can't begin to say what that's doing to the central nervous system and brain cells. It is pure insanity and a rush that we can't even begin to describe.

Back in the mid 90's when Stacker got involved with the energy drinks, which was long before Monster, Mountain Dew, Red Bull, etc. came out with energy drinks, it was all about those quick pick me ups before coffee or a grab and go. Stacker is now out of business but there's a ton of other energy drinks and energy bars that are loaded with caffeine that are dangerous, not only because of the amount of caffeine that's in them, but also because of the other drugs and inducers that's located in them. It's not only bad for your mental health, but physically as well.

Those are just some of the examples of caffeine and where it's found but in all honesty, caffeine is everywhere nowadays. It's always been around and will forever to be continued in our everyday lives.

When we look at the side effects of caffeine intake, there are some downsides of it, but then again there are some upsides. One of the downsides to caffeine intake is that it can cause dehydration. It can also cause rapid heart increase; which if you have high blood pressure to begin with, it can lead to trouble. It also causes a mild case of anxiety which can include the jittery feeling which includes having the shakes, a higher alertness than what your normally used to which can lead to a case of paranoia. It can also lead you to having to use the bathroom a lot more than you're typically used to.

The typical upsides of caffeine are again, it raises your alertness and creates less fatigue. It lowers the risk of heart disease (on a slow and steady usage). One of the biggest bright spots about caffeine intake is that it reduces the risk of depression and suicide. Even though some say that there is the possibility of low baby weight during pregnancy, there is no scientific evidence that says caffeine is harmful during terms.

So while this can be a controversial topic and there are people who will be willing to argue about whether caffeine is addictive, it's not so much that the drug in itself is; it's the causes and effects that are. It's the way that it makes you feel that can lead to the addiction.

When we look at the beginning of the book and determine what an addiction is, it's a habitual feeling. Do we find ourselves continuously looking for that jolt in the morning at work? That question can lead to the answer that yes, caffeine is addictive. Can we live without caffeine in our daily lives? Same thing, we can and there are some who go out of their way to avoid it.

For the sake of argument though, when dealing with addiction, we can say that it is addictive. Now is it the same kind of drug as alcohol, marijuana or cocaine? Absolutely not; but when dealing with drugs and stimulants, then the answer can be flipped around to a 100% yes. Do you have an addiction to caffeine? I think it would be safe to say that there isn't one person in our world who lives their life without being addicted to caffeine. In regards to battling this, there is no real answer to give. It is one of the healthiest drugs for us to consume, but must be done in small doses. If you do small daily doses, it can actually improve life.

Cocaine

Without distinction, one of the most lethal illegal drugs to ever been introduced to us comes in the form of a white powdery substance. Cocaine comes in many ways, colors, potency and names. It can be induced in many ways as well leaving us dangerously linked to this illegal drug. We are finding more and more users of cocaine are starting at a younger age as time passes us by.

Being someone who was at one time a chronic user of cocaine, I can tell you the effects this drug does are detrimental to your health in more ways than one. There are numerous ways that this drug can be done and each way is just as dangerous as the next. It can be inhaled, or smoked as most users choose to do. Then there's another way; which at first I didn't understand why someone would do it, and that's by putting a small amount in your mouth under the gums. While this allows the chemicals to go right into your bloodstream, this also causes rapid teeth loss as well as gum decay; regardless of how much you floss or brush your teeth.

I won't talk too much about the ways to use this drug because I don't want to promote the drug use, that's not what this book is about. If we're using the drugs, we already know how we feel.

If you are battling the addiction with cocaine, some relatives or friends might say it's too late to get away from the drug. But trust me when I tell you, it's not too late. You too can walk away from this drug without the usage of prescription drugs and without medical treatment. It's hard, and society isn't too keen on us who have battled our addictions, especially with cocaine. The withdrawals aren't fun, but if you follow my steps, you will be over this addiction.

First and foremost, find another person who used to be addicted to the drug and got away from it. As with the case in any drug, it is a lot easier to be able to find help, not a professional but another user who's been down the road that you're currently on.

Secondly, there are activities that you can do that will help you to be able to battle the addiction and get clean. Some of the things to do to occupy the mind and rebuild the health can be sports, playing cards, going to the gym or even going out for a walk. By doing this, you can and will build up a strong will and fight the addiction. It will take a while and will be a battle, but it will happen.

We can get into the multiple terms that's used for Cocaine, but I really don't want to touch base on every single topical name of coke. It's all bad news.

Third, find out which drug got you started on cocaine and get away from it. Some start with marijuana (which people always say that it's not a gateway drug) and I call you know what to it. The problem these days with drugs is that you don't know what you're getting and the dealers are putting more and more stuff into it and you chase that high. If we eliminate our gates, and start fresh, that will be one of the key factors to being able to beat the addiction of cocaine.

Lastly, take the money that you spend on your addiction and go to your bank and have it converted to pennies and put them in a jar. As crazy as this will sound, this does work just as much as going to the medical professionals. By the time you go through and count the pennies, re-wrap them, distribute them to get the cash, to get to the dealers, your mind is already over the addiction.

We can get out of Rock Bottom and defeat the battle of addiction to cocaine by replacing the chemical imbalance in our brain by keeping it occupied. The high is a short blast and cravings for the drug last between 5-16 minutes. We find something to do once the craving kicks in and trust me; we can and will get out of the hole and be able to beat this.

Drugs

In this chapter, we will discuss the random drugs and prescriptions that are given to us. Most of these are highly addictive and very dangerous not just because of the addiction, but also because of the harm that they cause to our bodies due to the side effects. It's very important that I say that while some of these drugs are needed as prescribed, it is very important that before being prescribed the drug, that the doctor knows **everything** that's going on, including if there's a history of depression in the family or if there's someone in the household that's either dealing with, or has prior dealt with drug abuse.

Ritalin is a chemical stimulant that's used to help with ADD, OCD, and ADHD as well as other problems in life such as Narcolepsy. If not taken as prescribed, or gets in the wrong hands so to speak, it can cause some of the following; blurred vision, hostility, seizures, chest pains where you feel you're having a heart attack, loss of appetite, sleep deprivation, and erection problems for men, to name a few. The one thing that strikes me with this is that it's used to help aid with narcolepsy, yet can cause sleep deprivation. So now you go to the doctor and they give you more drugs to combat the problem.

It's a never ending issue, or is it? The drugs Ritalin, Adderal and such doesn't cure the ailment, it only covers it, allowing the doctors to work with the insurance companies to be able to give us more drugs. The thing is, our bodies can combat issues on its own, providing that we allow it. The body is a wonderful thing and our immune system can defeat anything thrown in its path. So when given a drug to combat a sleep disorder, but yet can cause us to lose even more sleep, it's a head scratcher. We should allow ourselves extra time in the day to take naps, whether we're tired or not; even if it's a 20 minute power nap. It helps a great deal.

Reglan is one drug in particular that needs to be taken off the market. This drug is highly disputed and one could say that it's the safest drug to take, however the side effects are extremely severe. The drug is used to combat gastroparises, which is when one suffers from cleansing of the stomach. This drug when taken in long periods of time, more than 9-12 weeks, **can and will cause** essential tremors which leads to Parkinson's. There are too many people out there who have been given this drug that came down with it.

There are other natural herbs and other ways that you can beat the illness with instead of using this drug. When at the doctors, ask them for a list of ways without drugs or I could suggest using WebMD; the internet is a powerful tool these days and all the information out there is listed for free.

If the doctor prescribes Reglan or the medical name; metoclopramide, for whatever the case may be, for your own safety, seek another way. If you must still insist on using the medication that the doctor prescribes, as with **any and all** medication and prescription drugs, look up the drug name, the side effects, risk factor, and last but not least; long-term fatality rate.

Prednisone covers a whole field of medical issues that it can mask, however in itself; it is lethal. It's to be used in small doses as a cure for inflammatory diseases and help with things such as Asthma, MS, cancer, COPD and Poison Ivy/Oak exposure. While doctors give this out like its candy, it is detrimental with the side effects.

Most importantly, the short term effects have led to death. It causes anxiety, depression, and nervousness to name a few. Some of the minor effects of being on the drug are induced weight gain, diarrhea, et al. Major issues from this are as follows: Ulcers, aches and pains, loss of thought, and increased sugar in the blood.

Those side effects can be deadly to Diabetics due to raising glucose levels; it can also cause osteoporosis and glaucoma through long term usage.

Instead of being on prednisone, there are natural herbs and vitamins that can be taken to maintain health by being healthy. If you are on it short term, make sure it's short term; do not use this drug long term, it will kill you; and the death will be worse than can be imagined. If you've been on it for more than 6 months, seek immediate care as it's eating at you from the inside out and killing your organs.

Methotrexate is a drug that's not really known to men, but one of those drugs that are "needed" in life for chemo-therapy. This drug is administered in all types of cancer; and while the medical professional field says that it kills cancer cells, it also kills white blood cells and reduces the immune system through radiation. Does that sound safe? The human body is not meant to have radiation pumped into it and often times the body rejects it by making the patient sick.

If you're a patient who suffers from arthritis, the doctors are giving you this drug as well as prednisone. Again, prednisone is one of those drugs that should never be taken, and then you mix this drug with it, it **will** kill you. Some of the effects of methotrexate is as follows: Bone Marrow loss, Liver and Kidney toxicity, lung disease and the already mentioned lowered immune system; which opens the patient to a whole world of bacterial infections.

When we look at what methotrexate really is, it's a folic acid of Vitamin B; B7 to be exact. When we look at what the chemical effect does to our body, it goes to the neurological part of our body. Some can argue that we need **ALL** vitamins, but again, Vitamin B is one that should be excluded from our daily lives. It's only a temporary fix, it's deadly when used long term.

Coumadin, just like many of the other drugs that we have covered in this book and many of the others that are yet to come, is a head scratcher as to why the doctors would allow us to put this into our body. Granted, it *is* a blood thinner that can help rid us of blood clots, but over time, it is just as deadly. There are cases of where people have gotten a deep scratch and have bled to death.

All blood thinners should not be something that we look to induce into our lives. Blood thinners are a chemical composition that also involves a touch of rat poison, which is something that we shouldn't be putting into our body. It weakens our blood cells which in long term can and will cause strokes and heart attacks.

We can look for alternatives such as Vitamin C, which builds a wall around our red blood cells and allows for safer passage. We can take Vitamin E which is a healthy Vitamin that does prevent strokes.

Before we start putting these chemical composted drugs in our body, we really need to look and see what they truly do, and see the consequences of what's going on. Long before the medical field grew into a multi-billion dollar industry, there was natural vitamins and herbs; and there still here.

Cholesterol is definitely one of those items in our body that we can control without going to the doctors and smart physicians will tell you that. What they won't tell you is that when they put us on drugs just as Zocor, Colestid, and Questrain is that while it's helping your cholesterol, it's also opening you up to a whole new world of health issues for the duration of your life.

By being involved with these drugs, it raises your chances of having a heart attack by 42%. It also causes liver damage. It can also cause you to be nauseas, constipated and more. What these drugs do in the long haul is that they replace all the vitamins that your body needs to function in a proper working state, and gives it a chemical state that can release bile into your intestines and go so far as to give you types of blood diseases later in life.

By living a healthy life with a balanced diet with the proper carbohydrates, fiber, exercise and plenty of water intakes, our body will generate the type's and levels that we need to function. In this healthy way of living, we can also include Vitamin C. Vitamin C, which we all known is calcium is never harmful to the body. If you insist on going to the doctor to get medication, I can and will strongly suggest Niacin.

Prozac is one of those highly addictive drugs that are given to combat depression. Drugs like Prozac and Zoloft have often times created such mood swings in the user that it's unbearable to think of the acts that they have committed.

The problem with the drug is that it balances levels of serotonin in the brain with chemicals. Too much of these chemicals cause anxiousness, and obsessive behavior, as well as being agitated. Research has been done that 22% of the users have felt suicidal or have felt hostility towards others *while being on* Prozac.

The problem with society today is when someone feels depressed, the medical field is too quick to throw medication in their direction as if its candy, instead of offering alternatives such as vitamins, or telling people to get out and exercise. Depression is a state of mind that can be caused by a serious life event that doesn't need to be fixed by medication. We can beat depression by being around people and finding activities that will enlighten our mood, often times finding something that we will now enjoy and continue to do for the rest of our lives. Kids are committing suicide from doing this drug thinking that there's no hope; *KIDS.* This drug needs to be off the market.

Being someone who has dealt with depression and was prescribed medication after meeting a psychiatrist; the mood swings that I felt personally were something out of a movie. Friends and Family both noticed a Doctor Jekyll and Mr. Hyde personality. The thoughts of suicide were definitely there.

Then came my personal Rock Bottom and drug usage. I was searching for a different type of feeling and if it didn't work, I would've felt that there was no help. Mixing pills, doing drugs and drinking alcohol made for a terrible part of life that to this day, I regret living it. I don't necessarily regret some of the choices I made, but the path has followed, that thankfully someone helped me get better. Here I am almost 10 years clean and sober, living a much better life where there is no darkness. My life isn't perfect, but the choices I make now are far better off than they were.

My point is and why I'm putting this in with this chapter is simple; if we seek a better life and with a strong will, we don't need to feel down on ourselves. Our pain is only temporary and we don't need the burdens of a long term struggle with multiple types of addiction by using a pill. Find a hobby or something that you can enjoy and use it to your advantage. By being positive in life, only positive things will happen.

Diuretics are one of those drugs that can be healthy when used during a short term basis. When being prescribed, they are often used to help with hypertension. It may also be used to lower blood pressure. However, they also have long term effects that can be deadly.

They work by allowing the body to pass minerals, often times minerals that are beneficial to the body. The thing with Diuretics is it blocks the kidneys from being able to reabsorb minerals like sodium. This can be a good thing at times, but it has been proven to be fatal when taken on a daily basis. If there is a family tie to heart disease or congestive heart failure, this is one medication that shouldn't be prescribed to the user.

Instead of taking Diuretics, there are other ways that you can substitute and live a healthier life. You can drink clean, filtered water. You can also take and add magnesium and calcium to your daily food intake. You can also take Selenium, which helps in supporting the duties of the liver. Also, again, you can exercise or find a hobby that involves movement for 30 minutes to an hour a day.

It is through these ways that we can continue to live a happy and healthy life without the use of drugs.

Proscar is a drug that many men end up taking as they get elder. It is a drug that was created to help men with Prostate cancer and benign prostatic hypertrophy. What they're not telling you about the drug is that women are cautioned to not even handle the drug or have intercourse with men who are taking it due to it causing urogenital defects.

We know that Prostate cancer affects men and that it does take lives; roughly 50,000 men a year die from it. We also know that almost all men over the age of 65 have slow growing cancer cells in the prostate gland. The hard part is how do we keep them contained to one gland? If we do, then there is no issue other than just watching under the eye for a rapid change; which 9/10 times won't progress to anything severe.

We can take a natural herb at a young age (30-50) to help slow down this process, if not eliminate it completely. The natural herb is known as Srenoa. We don't need to go through surgery; we don't need medication and don't need radiation. All we are doing really is preventing the tumor cells from going into our other organs and naturally passing, instead of the cancer cells going through the blood stream causing us to have other issues in life that will kill us.

Glucotrol is a type of medication that's given to people who suffer from Type II Diabetes. It is a medication that is taken orally with a pill that's covered in sulfur. This medication as well as DiaBeta has been known to actually increase the possibilities of having heart attacks; and that's proven through scientific testing.

Diabetes has two forms; Type I is when the pancreas creates too little insulin and they will rely on insulin for the rest of their lives. Type II Diabetics rely on pills to help create insulin for the glucose level in their bodies.

However, when people have been placed on Glucotrol for long periods of time, it has caused headaches, hypoglycemia, gastrointestinal problems, and last but not least liver damage.

For those who want to get away from being insulin dependent or want to be healthy without the risk of becoming a diabetic, it is best to use vitamin B throughout your life; have a proper meal schedule and exercise. There are mixed reports about whether diabetes is a hereditary ailment and most women contract it while pregnant. Both of these are still under study and will be for a very long time. As said before in other parts, our bodies are wonderful and full of life.

OTC Drugs are drugs that are sold Over The Counter. I won't spend too much time in the book discussing these or what they do; but they can still be very dangerous to your health. They can be a temporary fix, which is what they are meant to do, but in the long run, not just the meds, but what's in them will do serious damage.

Drugs like Benadryl, Ibuprofen, Tylenol, Aspirin, et al. may provide a quick relief for a headache or a quick pain. We've all used them. However, putting them into a house where someone's addicted, it can reach for a scary situation. We all go through the phase of being addicted to medicine at this point. Headaches; how quick do we go for the medicine cabinet? Back pain; same issue?

Now; Let us look at the situation if you use alcohol in your life. These already can cause your heart rate to go up and vision to be distorted a bit, now drinking just makes it that much more dangerous. As with any drug, we can't mix them; let alone should be we taking them.

Regardless of how much pain we're in, we can practice meditation or use herbal plants in our coffee or tea to help. Too much of these meds can lead to an overdose, damage to your body, and even death.

Cough and Flu medication, including but not limited to syrup is something that we're all guilty of taking without knowing the true dangers that they possess. Many people like to self-medicate to try to get better; we've been trained to ever since an early age. While it may help by offering us a temporary fix, it also does harm to our immune system by lowering the white blood cells.

What some people don't realize is when doctors also tell us to maintain a proper rest schedule, it's so our bodies don't wear down and leave us viable to catch the common cold. We are also able to have magnetic water (as odd as that sounds) but that includes your soups and broths. They provide a huge amount of support to the body and make us feel good at the same time.

Another one of the best things that we can do on our own as we start to feel the symptoms of a cold coming on; is to start immediately on Emergen-C. It is a strong amount of Vitamin C which can be mixed with water and provides our body with enough to beat the bacteria. You can also use an olive leaf extract which is found in your local health or grocery stores. They fight the bacteria and provide enough strength for you to carry on through the day.

Calcium Channel Blockers such as Cardizem and Procardia are seriously dangerous to your health and increase your chances of getting heart disease by 63%. They do lower your blood pressure by blocking the entrance of calcium into the arterial cells in your heart.

One of the issues that we have with taking these meds is the simple fact that our body *needs* calcium. If you're having an issue with high blood pressure, there are other avenues to take that will help with bringing it down. But most importantly, we shouldn't be taking pills that slowly destroy our blood vessels and walls around the heart. Doctors prescribe this medication with no intent on letting the patient ever get off, meaning long term and a slow process of killing your heart.

I didn't mention the Beta blockers such as Inderal or Tenormin because when it comes down to it, they have the same cause; to weaken the heart. While on these types of medication, it causes loss of libido as well as the onset of fatigue, which is due to it lowering the blood pressure.

Instead of taking these pills, we can work on drinking more water, eating more fruit in our daily intake, and we can also take Immuzyme; which is a *natural* calcium channel blocker, not *chemicals.*

There is a whole list of other drugs that the doctors prescribe us that haven't even been mentioned. I'm not writing this book to start a war on drugs, nor am I in the medical field as mentioned time and time again in the earlier parts of the book. What I am doing in this, is trying to raise awareness that frankly put, whether prescribed or not, drugs are seriously bad to our health, even when induced for short periods of time.

When we look at what a drug is, it's a chemical substance. Some would argue that marijuana is a drug, and by rights it is, but others will argue that it's an herb which is partially true. We will get into that later in the book. Herbs are something that grows naturally without the use of chemicals. We can take herbal medicine and be healthy and live and long, prosperous life.

While I'd like to continue this chapter on drugs that are *prescribed*, I'm going to move on and talk about some other things in life that we can be addicted to; whether it affects us directly or indirectly. Just please, when going to the doctors when ill or suffering from an ailment, when you get your prescription and before turning it in, check to see what it is.

Fame

When we think of fame, we think of celebrities always trying to catch the eye of the paparazzi or using social media to reach their fans. This really isn't just about the celebrities. We are taught from a young age that we too seek the spotlight and that in itself is a rough road that we can be addicted to.

Whether it's at our jobs, or if we are involved in sports, or could even be a local "celebrity" we all seek that spotlight. We've all had that one boss who abuses their power a little too much. We all know that one guy in a recreational sports league that everyone knows has an ego the size of the team and they flaunt it. We know the person that's on a local community access channel that thinks they are better than everyone because they're on TV. We've seen reports of media personnel that break the rules to get a story. It's a general thing that we do.

The problem with seeking fame isn't so much that it's a big problem, because it's nice to be in that center of attention; it's the consequences of failure when the ride stops. It's the "I won't be like that" but then instantly turn into that person when we get back to it. It's the things we do to get back on top that can be bad to our health. How is this possible?

Let's say at your job, you've been given Employee of the Month or one step better; a promotion due to your work ethic and you picked up the type of work you're doing fast. You get along great with all your co-workers but now someone new comes in and they are now your responsibility. It's up to you to train them and get them to the level that you're at.

However, the thing is that they just aren't getting it as quick as you did. It's now up to you to decide; do I go to the boss and complain and it maybe gets them terminated, or do you give up on them in frustration and pass them on to someone else? Do you gossip about that person and make everyone not want to work with them? Do you make them feel bad enough about their performance that maybe they just give up and quit to go on to the next job?

We've all been in retail stores, grocery stores and even restaurants where this kind of stuff happens every day. As a consumer; better yet as a human being, we have to show compassion towards others. We have to allow ourselves to take a step back and not be in such a rush so we can help each other. Just because that person doesn't move or work as fast doesn't make them a bad person. We can help them get better by being better; not bitter.

We strive in our lives for that competitive edge and some of us excel at it better than others. That's what makes us so great, is our ability to try to perfectly execute what we do. In sports, we have our local heroes and some are lucky enough to make it to the big leagues. But those of us who aren't tend to be the "big person on campus" through our local rec leagues.

I personally am a member of the Professional Bowlers Association and remember when I got my card; it was one of the greatest things to happen in my life. Being the only one in my local center to have one, I have to say, it gave me a thrill and sort of a big chip on my shoulder. Then came the reality of other bowlers who were coming to me for advice. Knowing that I had the skill to compete, I decided that it was time to give back. I was one of them at one point in my life; needing help and asking for advice on what to do.

I mention the above because you see it in your local softball, basketball, bowling, darts, pool, etc. You see the "big dogs" get to a certain point then the ego subsides to a coaching point of view. It's like that with all athletes. There is no greater joy than being able to share the knowledge and help others achieve the success that we have. Whether you're a local athlete or a pro, help someone get to where you're at.

As I continue on this topic of fame, it strikes me that we always achieve and set the bar high for ourselves. It's not a bad thing, but when we do that we set ourselves up for failure.

When we say things like "it's my duty" or "I will be the greatest" it's a constant reminder that while we're setting ourselves up to be the best, we also reflect a bad image to others. When others look down on us, we feel the emotions and get conflictive. It's a part of our personal battles. It's great to be on top, but we have to remember what it felt like on the bottom.

When setting a goal, don't set it to be at the top. Set it for the middle and work your way up. We don't want to be that celebrity that's constantly trying to get in the news for their 5 minutes of fame. They have to continuously do something; anything; to continue to get the spotlight and most of the times, it's not a good spotlight.

We can make the spotlight shine on us for as long as we want if we do it progressively. We won't have that rapid fall to the bottom when we gradually go down. We can keep telling ourselves when things don't go right, which it can and will happen. All things happen. Help others and the fame by way of respect amongst your peers will be the greatest joy of all.

Fitness

One of the best things in our life that we can be addicted to is the ability to exercise and maintain a healthy lifestyle through fitness. When thinking about fitness, it's as simple as going for a jog/walk, going to the gym and working out through a proper regiment or swimming. We should spend 30 minutes a day at the minimum working out; it'll make our bodies last longer and feel greater.

On the flipside of the coin though, we all know and hear the horror stories of people who have gone to the extreme. It could be a case of doing steroids to get that extra weight, or a fitness model trying to cut weight and ending up getting too far. There is a natural way to do things, you don't need to do drugs or damage your body to get the look that's desired. We have to remember that we have a goal for ourselves and while I don't want to say "Settle with that look" it's okay to do that and maintain that level of your workout. The best way to get into fitness and maintain your exercise is when you get to the gym; they have pro trainers who get you started.

When we look at the way society has played a part in our lives today, it's a dangerous level with fitness. Let's divulge a bit.

We all see these big body builders out there who have had assistance to getting their look. There's ways to get that desired look, and to have the cuts without taking steroids. Not only is steroids a dangerous drug and severe health hazard, but in the end your body will fall apart. Look at the professional athletes who have gone on to either commit crimes, end up with a short career or even worse; dead. By eating balanced meals and a daily routine that focuses on certain targets of the body, you can look just the same without damaging the body.

The same statement can be made towards females; however they do a bit more of a struggle. Society today paints a picture of having to have that "perfect 10" look. From a young age, girls can get into serious health issues with trying to maintain a perfect look; something that's not needed. With a balanced diet and a healthy exercise plan, they too can have a perfect look.

We don't have to create other disorders and health issues to look like models, or on the covers of fitness magazines. Providing we spend the right amount of time at the gym, we load up on the proper carbs and proteins that our bodies need, we can be perfect with who we are.

Food

It's a bit ironic that we ended the last chapter by saying that we can enjoy a healthy lifestyle with the right balanced meals and then jump right into people who have dealt with food addictions. When we're addicted to certain types of food, yes it can pose huge health risks; other types of food, not so much.

We know from a very young age that there are the basic five food groups. We're also taught to have a balanced nutritional diet, though as the years go by we start to veer off the path and create our own. It is okay for us to want to snack and enjoy the finer things in life, it really is. But how much of what we eat in one sitting and the types of food we take in are what can cause us harm.

Not just through ingestion, but also the contents and chemicals that are used when the food is processed. Now not so much anymore, but there used to be GMO until mid-2000's when it was pulled off the market.

Let's not forget our snacks and sweets which we'll get into shortly but they can lead to other serious medical conditions as well as problems with our weight preventing us from living a healthy lifestyle. It's okay to snack on them here and there though.

Certain types of food have to be cleaned, cooked and prepped properly due to bacteria, which is general knowledge. You don't eat raw meat, or raw chicken. Seafood should be cooked and cleaned, though there is sushi, which is generally raw fish. Other types of food contain acids that have to be boiled out due to doing damage to your stomach. We also can have an addiction to fatty foods which can lead to clogs in arteries, even though the food may be what we feel we need. Foods that are high in cholesterol can be dangerous due to causing problems with the heart.

As previously mentioned, we have our sweet tooth and love snacks. It's a general thing that **all** of us enjoy and it's very easy to give into the temptation. Sometimes we overdo it and get that ill-fated stomach ache. Those who are diabetics sometimes use the snacks to hold the glucose at bay by snacking. It could be something as small as a chocolate bar or even Crackers with peanut butter on them. The issue with that is, when we do that and go to have our regular meal, it sometimes ends up being supplemented because our mind is saying that we're not hungry anymore. Ever cook a big meal and snack while doing it, then try to sit down at the dinner table? It's extremely difficult at times.

See; the thing is that it's not so much the food that we enjoy that can be the problem. When we talk about addiction, it can be a catch 22. We all know someone who has battled disorders in life and here's where the issues lay in wait and the majority of this is blamed on society; as with most cases when it comes to dealing with addictions.

Whether you're overweight or not at the ideal weight, we look at fast food and other meals as a quick grab and go. Whether you're overweight or under, we love our treats. The problem with society in todays' world is that if someone is overweight by 20 pounds, it's quick to judge. Now imagine telling a young kid that they are overweight. Now comes the mindset and depression of being viewed and bullied because of their build. Believe it or not, this has a life-long effect on the person for the rest of their life. Eating Disorders generally start at a young age and can continue for well over 24 years; if death doesn't set in before that.

As long as we keep a natural balanced diet and can get away with snacking accordingly, without going into excess or binge eating, we can be addicted to our favorite foods and not be in fear. This is one of the natural addictions that it's okay to have. We need food in our bodies to live, and live for what we enjoy.

Gambling

One of the worst addictions one can ever have is the addiction to gambling. This addiction has destroyed lives and has led some to go so far as committing crimes and even committing suicide. As things sit now, the addiction to gambling is a true heartbreaker and once you catch that bug; it is extremely difficult to step away from, especially when you try to chase that dream.

We're all guilty of trying to win the multi-million dollar jackpots even though we hear the horror stories of how winners have gone broke within a couple years. We all say that won't happen to us if given the chance. The problem is that we may say we're only going to buy one ticket, but as the jackpots climb, we started spending more on tickets and eventually find ourselves waiting for our next paycheck after finding out nobody won. The addiction doesn't end with just the multi-million dollar jackpot games.

We all know the big sporting events and the type of money that they can bring in when the bet is on the right side. With the technology now, you can find sites that allow you to place bets or take a short trip to the casinos to plunker money down on your favorite to win. Not to mention the horse races and et al.

It doesn't even have to be including those events. It can be the scratch games which are literally everywhere we turn. Scratch games are rewarding to an extent but often times create more losing tickets then they do winners. If you lay down $30 for tickets and win $20, when you are addicted, you will continue to play chasing the chance to get even; often times losing more. It's happened to too many people.

Casino trips can often lead to trouble. Being someone who has gone to the local casinos here in CT, we have a saying for card players; they come in with cars, go home on buses. It's not just with card players though. There are so many different types of games that it is just pure ridiculousness. You may hit once in a while, but more times than not the house wins. That's the way it's designed.

Sports gambling even at the recreational level tends to be a part of a topical mention here as well. How many times do we hear players say "How much you want to bet that this will happen?" It's constantly around us. When you're addicted to it, it just drags you right in. Bowling is the same way with side pots and all the other games, not to mention the card games that go on during the league. If you add drinking into the mix, a night of fun can now turn to an expensive night.

Ever look down at your gas gauge and knowingly drive by a gas station saying to yourself "I can make it to the next one" or "I don't have time to stop, I'll get it later?" Ever not buckle up; something that *everyone* is guilty of at one point in their life. With the latest push of no texting/talking while driving, we *still* see people push themselves to answer that call; saying "it's important, I need to take this." It's a gamble and its life.

I know I didn't get into too much detail here; trust me I didn't even scratch the surface. Gambling is one type of addiction that carries with us from the time we place our first bet all the way to our oldest day. It doesn't have to be with just gambling as far as cards, bingo and sports go. We always take a gamble within our life. It's how we're designed to go through life. This is not just an opinion as some would suggest; this is a *fact!*

We can get ourselves away from this addiction though. Most of it comes from habits that need to be changed. It will prove difficult because as they say, hard habits are tough to break, but as anything, it can be done. Our own willpower regardless of how weak we may seem at times, will give us the strength to get over this addiction. How is it possible? Let's look.

One of the easiest ways to break away from this addiction would be able to say to change some of the things we do in life. However, whether that may be possible it still won't affect the outcome. There are still things in life that can and will lead this addiction disease to continue in our lives. Again, I'm not talking just about the gambling through the lottery, I'm talking about the gambling addiction with our ways of life.

As I mentioned on the previous page, we constantly take chances and risks by gambling with our lives. We can be better prepared by knowing what the risks are and trying our best to prevent them. We can take the extra couple minutes in our lives to make sure that we are practicing safety.

We all know that we need our phones in case of an emergency, but especially those of us who are younger in age; we can start by putting our cell phones in the glove compartment when we first get in the vehicle. As dumb as this may sound, this will help in a couple different ways. By the time we reach over to get it out, especially at a high rate of speed, it leads to dangers. By doing this, it forces us to have to pull to the side of the road or better yet, wait until we get to our destination. Nothing is as important as your life, not even a phone call or a text from a friend saying hi.

When we're dealing with the addiction of gambling when it comes to sporting events and the ill-fated dream of winning the lotto, there's a couple of different things that we can do to win against this battle.

First and foremost, when it comes to the lotto it's okay to dream big. If you remember what we talked about earlier in the book, we don't want those dreams and goals to be so far away from us that we set up for failure. How many people do you know that won big on the lotto? Very few of us do know many people and chances are the biggest that was won was around a thousand dollars on a slot machine.

We're not focusing just on the slots, but even those of us who have a hard time dealing with scratch tickets; we get them from the same location because we feel "lucky there." To combat this, we can switch our route and avoid that place altogether. On the flipside of this coin though, you will still pass other places that sell lotto tickets and in today's day in age, all types of lotto are everywhere. You can't even go to a bar and enjoy a cocktail without seeing a lotto machine there doing some type of game, including Keno. It's not possible. To break away from this, there's a mental picture that you can do for yourself.

The next time that you're thinking about going on a splurge for the scratch tickets or even for the lucky lottery tickets, picture yourself going to the bank.

You can go to your own bank and put a $50 bill on the counter and asking them for change in coins. Now take that change home and put $10 of it away in a place that you'll remember where it's at. Take the other change, open it up and put it in a bowl. Now go to your bathroom and coin by coin, throw it in your toilet. For every two dollars that you throw in there, flush the toilet. You might get lucky and see some of the change come back to you. You might also clog the drain, but that's the chances you'll take. As dumb as this may sound, there are a few people who were professional gamblers that got away from the addiction by doing this.

You can also take and give the money that you worked for away. You don't know if the next person is suffering from gambling too so you might say "well hey, that won't work." Trust me when I tell you, buying a stranger a cup of coffee does wonders not just for yourself, but for others as well. Remember a few years ago when we had the "Pay It Forward" craze? It's still here and you can continue it. This part works and will easily help you get over the addiction.

Habitual Lying

When dealing with addictions, not everything involves drugs and alcohol. There are other types as we have previously mentioned and more to come, including this one which is a big one for a lot of people in life. We all know that one person who is a story teller; we may not know their motives or what causes them to have to do this, but there are people in this world who are addicted to having to live their life surrounded by lying.

We can start out by saying that either we have found ourselves in a jam and have told a lie. The snowball effect starts to happen from there. You have to tell another lie to cover it, then another and the pattern of habitual lying has formed. The problem with habitual lying is unless you have a strong memory and can remember why the lie was formed and the original lie, there's always going to be that one person waiting in the wings to try to catch you on it. One small lie; or fib, doesn't make you a bad person and won't get you the reputation of being a liar. It's when it continues to happen that your trust goes out the window and people begin to back away when getting in a conversation with you.

In life for some, most of us, our reputations mean a lot and can either make or break us. If you're involved in a professional field and have clients, you will get more clients when they're able to trust you due to passing of word of mouth. As soon as the terms "liar, unreliable, unstable, etc." get passed around and it involves you or even worse; your business, nobody will want to hire you.

Take two restaurants that both sell the exact same things for the exact same prices. We can even begin to say that they'll be sitting across the street from each other. For sake of argument, let's say that we're going there for chicken. They both say that they serve 100% real chicken, but when you look up the reviews on the restaurant, you find out they aren't. Upon further reviews, you find that the restaurant has horrible staff problems, it's not clean and the bathrooms are a mess.

Which of those two businesses are you going to support now? The one that is getting through by lying and giving out false facts about their business or the one that's loaded with 5 star reviews and everyone tells you about all the time? Naturally, we'll choose the one with the good reviews.

Granted, there are some fields where being a liar can get you some pretty good money. Lawyers who argue for the defense, some doctors in the medical field when they give you meds that they know you shouldn't be on, some investors and a lot of bartenders, and last but not least; politicians.

I'm not saying any bartenders in general, but there are some who take their rings off or disperse knowledge of a relationship so they can get better tips, which is understandable to an extent. It's also been known to happen in the restaurant industry so it's not limited to just bartenders.

The problem arises when you have to ask "where does the lie begin and where does it end?" As with anything, if we can identify the problem, we **can fix the problem.** It's easy to say just to not lie, but even in our youth, we've been taught that it's okay to fib. But as our times change and we get older, it's tougher to break habits once their formed. We can blame it on stress, alcohol, and such but it still doesn't change the problem. To fix this, we really just have to start to look at ourselves and ask if this is the way we want to live. If this is how we want to be treated and would we respect the person doing it to us? Can we break the habit and get back on top? Most definitely we can.

Heroin

When deciding to write this book, it was with a goal in mind; to raise awareness on addiction and some of the most lethal drugs involved that people turn to when at Rock Bottom. Even though Heroin is considered an opiate, this drug needs to be separated and dealt with on its own. We will deal with opiates later in the book, as you saw earlier.

Heroine was originally discovered in the late 1800s and was used not just recreationally but medically. To this day, some countries allow the usage of heroin by prescription for people who are addicted to it. Originally derived for a pain medication, users feel a sudden rush of happiness and can be become addicted to the feeling they get from the drug.

The question one can ask is why do people need a drug to get that particular feeling? The answer to that can be a simple one but in the same notion, it can be difficult to answer. When it comes to being an addict, we get multiple thrills at a time. Not only through the usage of the drug, and the effects that the drug supplies us, but also because of how we received the illegal drugs. It's a thrill for us to not only use the drug, to fulfill our craving for the high, and break the law to get our drug of choice.

While we may be addicted to the effects that it gives us that lasts anywhere between 3-6 hours, the long term effects are detrimental to our health. Not only do we become addicted to the feeling that we get from it, but it can also cause long term pneumonia, an infection in the valves of the heart, collapsed veins and other illnesses including HIV; if done with a shared needle. It's not just the fact that we can get sick that causes this to be a bad drug; it's that the medical field likes to say the only way to cure this addiction is with the use of another drug.

That may be partially accurate but with anything; why are we going to use one drug to take care of another drug? One of the drugs that are given to us to get over the adverse reactions of Heroin and other opiates is methadone; which is something else we'll discuss later.

In all honesty, if you're battling an addiction with heroin, if you're in the early stages you can definitely beat the addiction from within. Even if the addiction has already set in, you can beat this on your own. Just like with alcohol, we need to seek guidance. Find something that you enjoy other than the drug and do that. It may sound hard, but there's other ways.

Whether you believe in spiritual power or not, one of the key ways to beat the addiction is to give your strength to the higher power. By picking up the book when you have the craving will decrease the chance of you using again by an average of 38%. It may not sound like much of a chance, but the more you do that, the more you give yourself a chance at life.

Something else that you can do is to activate your networking and reach out to others who have suffered through the addiction. I'm not talking just N.A. or any support groups like that. I do believe that they work, but by talking to another addict and finding out what they did to get and stay clean will help you down your path.

If you incorporate these steps and have **faith in yourself**, then you can beat the addiction. With some drugs they say that it's not wise to try to beat it by being alone, but you can do anything you want as long as you're willing to put the effort in. You can do anything you want if you feel the desire and need to be clean. Heroin addiction is one of the toughest to kick, but if you look at the alternative and remind yourself that it's not the way, you can kick it. Especially if you have kids, they need you to be there for them. No kid should ever have to bury their parents.

Internet

Technology in today's world is so far advanced that this is the easiest one for us all to admit that we're addicted to. No matter where you go, or what you're doing, the internet is setting you up to be a victim. It's very easy for the internet to take over our lives and it doesn't matter who you are or what profession you're in, your life is surrounded with an addiction to the internet. How do we get around this tough addiction though? What are some of the prime examples of having an internet addiction? Let's take a look.

In today's society, it's natural for us to carry cell phones and no matter where you go there's wifi. Most businesses that have wifi turned on, supply two servers; one private and one public. The public one is for patrons to use for browsing, whether it's the business site for coupons, specials, menus etc. The private server is designed for wait-staff and personnel. If you're using a public server and doing online banking, it's very easy to make yourself vulnerable for someone to get access to your information. With a public server, it's just that; it's open to anyone and everyone that can get on that signal. We've all heard reports of people being scammed and purchases that they didn't make; this is part of the reason.

Sticking with that side of the ball for a minute, there's another issue with the internet that has to do with businesses. If someone knows what they're doing, they can get a scanner app in their phone which doesn't even have to come in contact with you, only a matter of 4 feet, where they can get your credit card information that's in your wallet, upload it to the internet at home and max out your credit cards, all within a matter of a 20 minute meal. It has been done to people in the past and will continue to happen.

We've all been fond of using our fancy phones for texting while driving or answering that phone call that can wait while drinking our coffee or tea and driving. Not only do we put ourselves at risk for severe harm, but we're also endangering others. Luckily, they are trying to prevent it from happening and are now making it a law to where you can't use your phone while driving. It's not so much that but if you're on a road trip and need to change your GPS to update the route, or feel like you missed a step and go to look at the phone, that creates a whole separate issue. We can't really expect the cops to enforce this issue because in reality; the true problem is; we continue to do it because we see cops doing the same thing. But this is side-tracked, let's get back on point.

The internet can be a wonderful thing to be addicted to. The internet is and forever will be known as the information super-highway. I love using the internet to look up medication and use it constantly to get information on things when I'm out, or if traveling and need a number or want to look up an establishment, Google comes right up and away I go.

If you love to cook, there's literally a million different websites that you can go to and find that recipe for that awesome meal for entertainment. Just about every single recipe; including the infamous family recipes that you made are somewhere and people can offer insights and different variations.

If you love entertainment, you can find out what's hot and what's not in all fields of media. Whether you listen to music, watch TV, sports, movies or even do some book reading, it's all on the internet and just about all of it's available for FREE! Who doesn't love free stuff? Even for stuff that you have to pay for, there are other sites out there that you can get it for free.

Just be careful because some sites have click-bait ads; which are loaded with viruses and info stealers that will scan your hard drives for credit card numbers and important information.

One of the greatest tools of the internet is the amount of information available. I know I said that before but being addicted to the internet is not a bad thing. If it's a rainy day, look up a topic on something and read. Use the knowledge to your advantage. If there's anything that you're on for medication wise, you really should look up what it is that you're taking before taking it.

If you love video games, same as everything, there's a ton of options and most are free. Nowadays, computers and phones or tablets come pre-installed with games and you can just add on to them. However, we will discuss video games later on because there are some issues that need to be talked about.

The only real issue is that you have to proceed with caution when using social media. Granted, it's a wonderful thing to connect with those that aren't near or to meet new friends and family, but it's also been one of the key components of identity theft and scams galore. Be careful and know who you're talking to.

You see, if you're at Rock Bottom, one of the greatest things you can do is to have an addiction to the internet. It will do a wonderful thing to you. If you're isolated and feel the need to escape, you can. If you're feeling sad and need to get joy, you can.

Marijuana

Better known as cannabis, marijuana serves many purposes. Some are good but most are bad. One of the biggest and toughest addictions one person can have is to marijuana. It has been a topic of discussion for many years and will continue to be one as far as whether it's considered a "gateway drug." Though now most states in America have made it legal to have through medical usages, it's still a touchy subject.

When smoked straight, yes it does have its benefits and slows certain medical processes down. It's been said to help with cancer patients and people who have glaucoma, as well as help those with Parkinson's disease; although, I do have a problem with saying that it's a safe drug. No drug is or should ever be considered as a "safe drug." A drug is exactly that; a drug. And yes, drugs are addictive and can kill.

As being someone who started using my first drug with marijuana, I found myself getting bored over time and starting to mix it with other drugs. As an addict always looking for that greater rush, it's what we do. From there the downfall continues to experimenting with other drugs and the addiction grows. Before you know it, now there are more problems than what was originally had.

Even though there have been no reported deaths due to smoking marijuana, it does have some major side effects that go along with it. The side effects can vary on a person to person basis and can last anywhere from 20 minutes up to 2 hours. These side effects include mass anxiety, disruption of thought process, relaxation and increased heart rate.

It can be argued about your motor skills being affected, such as in going out to drive a car. First and foremost, as mentioned you're in a relaxed state of mind or as some would get a case of nonstop laughing. Being behind the wheel of a 1 ton vehicle may decrease your chance of speed as well as decrease your chance of stopping if needed to quickly. Add alcohol to the mix as most do, and it's a deadly combination.

If you're a new smoker, the best advice I can give you is to change your scenery to get away from this. The addiction to this drug will make you chase a stronger and longer high, leading into using other drugs. Talk to other users and you'll find out. Medical studies will tell you otherwise, but that's because the professional field and the government now makes money off you. So now they get double the money for your hard work and your recreational usages.

Meth

Methamphetamine or better known as meth is one of those drugs that have been around since the late 1800's. Originally prescribed for ADHD, it has since taken a turn for the worse and is now used as a party drug. Meth comes in many shapes and forms, most noticeably as crystal meth. However, in the fight against drugs and being a former addict, there's other ways for users to get meth, including over the counter; believe it or not. We'll touch on this in a minute.

Meth in itself is a highly addictive drug and also one of the strongest drugs that lead to the user going through bad withdrawals. When we look at what meth does to the user, it creates a high level of alertness and a boost in energy, but it also causes rapid weight loss. When a user does meth at a higher dosage, it can cause seizures, violent behavior and will damage your Central Nervous System. By doing meth, it can raise your risk of getting Parkinson's disease by almost 70%. Overdosing on meth can and will lead to death. Some of the early signs of an overdose include painful urination, aches, rapid heartbeat, and cold sweats. If you or someone you know is experiencing any of these signs, get to the nearest medical treatment center immediately.

Before we get into crystal meth and the dangers of it, there is a need to discuss a type of meth that's being sold currently over the counter. It's found in most of your nasal decongestant sprays and it's known as levomethamphetamine. It may not be as addictive as regular meth, but it's still meth and still dangerous when used too much. This will show up in urine tests and if you go for a physical, which is why some athletes get caught with this in their system, including pros.

If you know someone in your family or friends that are in the early stages of Parkinson's disease, the doctor's will prescribe a pill that has a chemical composition of meth in it, that pill is called Selegiline. This medication also comes in a patch form for ADHD. Your family pet will sometimes be prescribed Anipryl for Cushing's disease. I'm mentioning these so you know what to look for.

Crystal meth is the most common way that users and addicts get involved with meth. This is the most potent form and highly addictive. Not only that but it's also the most destructive in more ways than one can possibly even imagine. Not only does it destroy people on the outside and physically, but this drug can and will rip a family to shreds. This next page will discuss some of the signs and dangers of crystal meth.

Let's take a look at some of the dangers that users can and will experience during their life of crystal meth use before experiencing death from the addiction or a straightened out life.

Extreme weight loss and anorexia are the most common in female users. The meth usage doesn't allow their bodies to get the required nutrients that are needed to get back into shape and keep up.

Crime is also at an all-time high right now in the United States and not saying everyone is on meth, but Robbery and theft are two key things that are involved with addicts. They run into financial ruin and eventually have to have that unlimited supply of money to support the habit.

Tremors and convulsions can start in the body. With doing crystal meth, your body gets confused by the signals that it's getting and goes into a state of chaos. This will cause your body to start twitching and having some very violent issues with tremors. This can also lead to users developing Parkinson's disease at one point in their life.

Broken relationships are one of the key aspects that an addict can and will experience. Meth becomes your first priority, so things won't end just due to mood swings that are present, but through neglect.

Meth mouth is one of the other physical things that will happen to users. Even after the user has found the straight path and able to get clean; the process has already started since day one. The gums and teeth become weak and start to fall out. You can floss every day, but with meth it's a guarantee to happen.

Daily breathing and other respiratory issues will also be a sign of things to come for users. Due to what it does to your lungs and upper chest cavity, it will kill you from the inside out. It will also cause you to have a feeling as if you're having a stroke.

Last but not least, on top of the others that haven't been mentioned is the ability to perform during sexual contact. The user experiences an appetite for it during the early stages of meth use, but within a matter of 2 years, the ability to have an erection and perform diminishes.

Addicts can start out as the nicest people in the world, they can be family or friends and you may not know that they have an addiction to meth, but again; the signs are there. This drug is not one to mess around with. I'd like to say that it can be beat on one persons' own will, but sadly this drug is too dangerous to try. Rehab facilities and former users are the best.

Morphine

Morphine is another opiate that I feel has to be separated from that category. Taking morphine by itself won't kill you, it's the overdose or immense side effects that will. Morphine however can lead to trouble due to its highly addictive feeling and relief of pain. Morphine attacks the Central Nervous System and is often used for labor, accidents, and chronic pain.

Even though it's often given through IV at the hospital through doctors' care, it can also be shot with a needle or taken orally through pill form. The relief usually takes 10 minutes before it kicks in and can last anywhere from four to eight hours.

The key problem with using morphine is the sensation that one gets from using it. Like with any drug, the user gets adept to that feeling and soon wants that release for all types of pain. When that happens, the body becomes prone and the blood pressure continues to drop setting them up for organ failure, tissue damage, being tired and weak all the time, a feeling of loneliness as well.

The feeling may be good at times, but this drug is exactly that; a drug. You don't need to be medically induced with drugs to relieve pain, especially opiates. We'll discuss this again later in the opiates chapter.

Nicotine

Considered the most addictive drug, where would we be in this book without discussing nicotine. Nicotine and caffeine go together when it comes to having a morning pot of coffee. Nicotine and alcohol go together when out with a group of friends doing the bar hopping scene. In case you haven't figured it out yet, we're talking about cigarettes; though nicotine is found outside of cigarettes.

Smoking is a bad habit; take it from someone who does it. It's not just based off what it does to your health, but the vehicle you drive and the clothes you wear reap the smell of tobacco. The house you live in will smell of the tobacco that's in the cigarettes. Nicotine is a stimulant but also works as a relaxant. In the immediate seven seconds after a puff of a cigarette, the nicotine passes from the lungs to the brain and triggers the receptors. So if you're under stress from work or an activity or something in life is even bothering you, being a smoker, you automatically reach for that cigarette and it calms you down.

They say nicotine in small doses isn't deadly, hence why when you try to quit smoking they give you the nicotrol gum or the patch. That may be true, but instinct kicks in because it's not enough.

Nicotine is just like every other drug in this book. It gives you that feeling that we as addicts try to chase, and regardless of how we get it, we succeed. How much is too much? When we look at it that way, we can find out that nicotine *is a poison*. The real answer is 40mg of nicotine can be harmful, however there have been reports of higher numbers, numbers over 600mg.

Some of the side effects of nicotine include a raised heart rate and blood pressure, a spasm in the lungs, enlargement of the heart, headaches, sleep disturbances, and cancer.

It's not just the nicotine that's the problem. Yes, nicotine is a highly addictive drug that's found in cigarettes. We can say we're quitting, especially with the price of the cigarettes continuing to climb. We can say we're quitting because it's getting to be a hassle if we're sports fans, or to the point to where the government is saying you can't even have a cigarette in your car. It's easy for them to want to regulate our life, but it's not easy for us to walk away from something that we as addicts do. It's easy for the pharmacies and doctors and government to push medication on us so they can make money, but we will have our vises. You can quit on your own, I just don't know how to say it.

I can say that when trying to quit cigarettes, from what others have told me; you can try some of the following:

They always say that chewing gum works. It might work because it gives you something to put in your mouth and to resist the craving.

They used to say at one time to put a toothpick in your mouth. The farmers of the old days used to put a piece of hay in their mouth. It's been said that this satisfies the mind of wanting that cigarette in the mouth.

They say that the patches work. This could be true but I know on a personal level, and I've been a smoker for 19 years; that a patch will not resist my craving.

The problem that I face with millions of other people with nicotine and tobacco is I need that cigarette to go with my morning coffee. The job field that I work in is stressful and that break calms me down; not that I'm the flippy type. I hate driving in traffic and my nerves go through the roof, so when in a traffic jam, I reach for that cigarette to calm my nerves. It's how we handle things as a smoker. It's that we started the addiction at a young age and now it's a part of our daily life with how we handle certain things.

Opiates

We have already spent some time covering the drugs that are involved with opiates but there is a lot more types of other drugs out there that are in this particular field. I wish I could cover each and every drug that comes from this alkaloid chemical compounded drug. The drug actually comes from an opium poppy plant that's grown through the world, and illegal to grow here in the United States unless authorized by the Federal Government.

Some of the drugs that come from opiates but not limited to include; hydrocodone, oxycodone, heroin and morphine. Most of these we already spent some time covering. The thing that we're going to spend most of the time in this chapter is if you're already addicted or know someone who has an addiction to opiates, how we do get that turned around? How do we prevent a loved one from eventually overdosing and going into cardiac arrest? How do we prevent someone who replaces a feeling of pain and being lost to showing them a world of better living without being in pain?

There is a battle and it can be done both by the addict on their own account and with help from others. It's not an easy battle, but it is a rewarding one.

First things first, the hard part is getting through the withdrawals. The withdrawals do last anywhere from a week to three weeks. Those can include anything from feeling weak, nauseous, muscle aches and a real sense of human pain. The last one is a very important one because now the parts of your body that didn't hurt; will hurt due to the mind sending signals to get the pain relief.

As we're going through the withdrawals and starting to get into a healthy living without the use of drugs; we can start to work on a recovery plan. In our recovery plan, we need to get rid of the self-shaming and the cycle of guilt. This is a key element due to the feeling of being addicted to a pain killer. There are programs out there that involve other addicts who have found recovery through "Strength in numbers." Let's face it though, as an addict we aren't very straight-forward with others about our addictions. We put that wall up because of the guilt. You can share with others about what's ailing you and they can help you become more vocal. By doing that, you just might be saving another persons' life. You can also remove yourself from the situation. Lastly and definitely most importantly, avoid going to anywhere you went before to get the opiates, and do one day at a time.

Sexual

I'm not going to spend a lot of time in the book talking about the addiction that some people may have to sex, although it does have to bear mentioning because it is a problem with todays' society.

What we do behind closed doors is one thing, and frankly put; it's none of anybody's business. The hard part about society is the way that they pre-judge people for activities. It can be anything from a late night romp to the way someone dresses; judging from society.

There was a time not too long ago when it was okay to dress how you saw fit. It was okay to dress sexy and cut loose for a night out on the town. Hell, it was promoted everywhere you looked. It was at one time okay to even do stuff in public, (don't believe me, look it up). With the way things are today and the way that people get labeled for every little thing that they do or don't do, it's ridiculous.

Part of this has to do with people being mentally sick and being sexual predators; people who spend too much time looking at internet porn sites; people who use internet for images; people who watch Hollywood act things out then try to take and feel it's okay for them to do it.

It's a sick world that we live in and will only continue to get worse. Things have to get worse before they can get better. But what causes one to be addicted? Is it the pleasure or the pain?

With the case of sexual predators and child molesters, they say that it's a mental disease or it's based on revenge. Part of that can be true; but another part of that can be debated and will forever be debated.

The majority of though, can be blamed on society. Granted, the ways some of the kids these days dress don't leave much for one to imagine, but it's the style these days. When I was a kid, guys dressed professionally and girls wore slacks. If they wore a dress, they were sent home and told to change. This was in the 90's and in a public school. Then came the boom of the younger generation. It was okay to wear short shorts again, low cut tops and mini-skirts made their return. Colleges around the country we're blindly hosting parties that encouraged acts. Guys became more worried about "the notches on their belts" more than the grades they were getting. Girls were the same. Maybe this is just a trend that will fade away or it will continue to get worse. Nobody knows the answer to that question, and won't ever be known.

Self-Importance

Self-importance is one thing that it's okay to be addicted in a sense. It's okay to walk around with a large ego; providing you can back up what you say. It's okay to be protective of things that are happening around you. It's okay to know the surroundings that are involved with your life. It's okay to know what your value in life is.

Where it's not good to be addicted to your "value" is when it gets to be too much. It's very easy for some of us to be caught up in ourselves. Look at some professional athletes who have risen through the ranks to be on top; then completely forget where they got their start. It happens all the time. Then there are others who have remained humble and gave back to the fans and community where they got their start.

You see other people in the corporate working world who use the power of position to their advantage and completely destroy their outside world without knowing it until it's too late. We've already discussed this happening earlier in the book, but it's an everyday occurrence. It doesn't even have to just be in the corporate world, it can be on the local level.

Dealing with self-importance, it's important that wherever you are, whatever you're doing, that you stay humble and gracious for what it is that you're doing. We all start somewhere and some pick things up faster than others. It's during this time that we remember to help others; by doing that, we gain self-worth that will last a lot longer than our height of an ego.

Speaking of ego, it's okay to have one if you can back up what goes with it. Lots of times people claim to be the greatest at what they do since sliced bread; that can be true for a certain time. Other times though, someone or something comes along and can knock them down off that pedestal faster than they rose to the top. It's important that we keep our ego in check.

It's okay to be arrogant without being cocky. We can be proud of whom we are and what it is that we're doing and flaunt it. Just remember that image that it'll look like to others. Just remember that time will eventually come where you're the one that's on the other end of the gloat and see how it'll feel.

Be who you are, be proud of what you are, and stay where you're at. Normality is a wonderful thing without being overly proud. Life is great when we can all share the value of life, instead of being ignored.

Shopping

We all see those crazy deals as we walk through stores, search the internet, and gallop through the grocery stores. Sometimes it can be fun to catch the great deals, and other times it can be frustrating especially when the store is out of stock. It can be a thrill for whatever reason and will always entice us to keep going. Especially when it's for stuff that we don't really need but we see it and it ends up going home with us. It's happened to all of us.

The thing that happens the most with shopping is what some may call an **impulsive buy.** It's when the stores put something out that they had on sale cheaper previously but you didn't need it then but do now. An impulsive buy is a problem when you're addicted because it can lead to financial debt as well as cluttered closets and spaces. It can lead to an addicted being labeled as a hoarder. It can happen to everyone and believe it or not; it has happened to all of us at one point or another. You don't have to be rich or poor to become an impulsive buyer. We can program ourselves to say "it's only just this once," but how many times have we all said something along those lines?

Sometimes in life we sacrifice the things we need for the things we want; that can be dangerous.

Take going grocery shopping for an example. Let's say it's a weekly thing and that you spend an average of $150 per family. By the time you go through the store and get your bare essentials that are needed in the basic food groups, you could easily top the $100 price tag. Now as you're walking through the store, you start throwing items in the cart that really aren't needed but that you want; could be anything from sweets to additional snacks for the kids or work. Next thing you know, you're up over the limit that you normally spend. We're not even getting into the part if you have a smoker and drinker in the household.

At the end of the week or month, that extra $30-60 a week adds up and now you're in the hole. If you writes checks or pay with a credit card and there's no money but still the need for groceries, now's it's an issue of going over-limit or writing a bad check and having to pay fees. Those fees add up especially when it continues to happen, or having to go to different stores due to not wanting to go back to the same store until the money is there. Remember, most banks charge anywhere from $20-40 per check. Most credit cards have a $35 over-limit charge **plus** interest. Now factor in that there are other things that you need throughout the month, but can't get without money.

I used the grocery store example for a reason as opposed to say; a department store. This happens more with grocery stores because it's easier to overspend there more than it is at a different store. We won't even get into stores that are considered big-box chains such as Wal-Mart where you can get clothes, groceries, electronics, etc.

It is really easy to find yourself in serious trouble when you become addicted to shopping, and it's one of the easiest addictions to have. It can be one the easiest to overcome as well. The power of self-will can help you escape the **Rock Bottom** of financial ruins and get some more money in your pocket with enough savings.

First way to beat this as mentioned previously, is the part of reminding yourself of what you want versus what you need. Only get the things that you need; tell yourself that you're not going to get what you want and continue to walk past it. Skip that aisle and ignore the front displays. Being involved in retail, those are placed there for a reason and it's not because they're on sale. If you do this enough for a couple weeks, you'll see some extra money showing up in the account that can be used for a later shopping trip and at the end of the month, if you want to splurge a bit, you can.

Second way to beat it is to cut back on your spending limits. Instead of saying "I'm going with $150, cut that down to $125 or less." If you go shopping during the week, you can even go to the bank and go shopping with cash, which will force you to use a set spending limit as opposed to free will.

I'm not going to say to change your eating habits, but that can make a difference too when shopping. They say in polls that the average family goes out to eat 3 nights a week and going out to eat isn't cheap anymore. You used to be able to feed a family of 4 for less than $25. With the cost of food rising, that family meal is now close to $50. Multiply that by the amount of nights you go out, and that can lead to unexpected costs. You can have the same food by having a home cooked meal and save nearly 70% of the cost; and spend time together as a family at home. By doing a home cooked meal, you can get the whole family involved and make it fun.

I'm not saying that you should cut everything out of life when it comes to shopping because we do all have needs. It's just that we have to learn our patterns and spending habits. We can work on them and be able to save money so we can eventually get the things we want in time.

Speed

In this chapter, we're not going to spend too much time talking about the narcotic known as speed because it's already been covered a bit due to it being another name for methamphetamines. We will spend most of this chapter talking about the infamous people that we come across everyday who are in a hurry to get nowhere fast. We'll talk about those who have to get the adrenaline rush of speeding and breaking the law.

We come across these people on a daily basis; we might even be one of them. We always see the people weaving in and out of traffic at free-will narrowly missing cars as they are at full speed. What does this actually get us when we come across traffic on the highway? It may be a satisfying feeling and the chance to be a risk taker, but with those risks come high chances of encountering fatal accidents. Not just on dry pavement, but if the roads are wet it can and will cause hydroplaning. We all know as drivers that we have blind spots that we think is free to move into and now someone comes flying into it, it can lead to a severe accident. We can say wrong place at the wrong time. But we can also say were we at fault or were they? These are all things we find ourselves doing too.

Gone are the days when we try to leave the house five minutes sooner to get to work. Gone are the days when we would be at work anywhere from ten minutes to a half hour early. It's not because we love our job that much, but it's about being on time and accounting for traffic. We can only control what we do, not others. When you factor in the speeding that we do to try and pick up lost time, with the stop for coffee or possibly calling your job to say you're late, now it's distracted driving at a high rate of speed. You may get away with it here and there, but at one point in your life, it will catch up with you.

In today's generation of drivers and with more cars being on the road, it just adds that much of an element to the dangers. Again, we can't control others, but we can control ourselves. Traffic these days are at an all-time high and will continue to grow. As there are more vehicles on the road and less space, it becomes an issue of where to go. We can get to our destination actually faster by not speeding, but going with traffic. We can get to our vacations safer without going faster and it'll save in the wallets. Imagine yourself driving down the road with a family in your vehicle driving at 90mph. Is that really how you want to see yourself and risk the lives of your family?

Sports

When it comes to being addictive to being active in sports, it's not so much a health issue nor is it a problem. It's good for the vascular to stay active as we mentioned in fitness. The parts that can be a problem is leaving you open to injuries. Injuries that at a young age will catch up to you as you get older. We have to remember that as we get older, parts of our body begin to wear down regardless of how physically fit we are. The games we play in sports will also play a part in what type of injuries we sustain.

I'm not going to get into the physical part of what can happen; we're already aware of it. It's the chances we take when we get physically involved in something. Just about every sport there is, even ones that are considered a hobby can lead to an injury; including fishing and yes; even a game like poker.

We can also find ourselves in a heap of trouble by the sports team that we're rooting for. Not just because alcohol could lead a part of the trouble, but some of the rivalries are so intense that people forget about courtesy and decide to get in brawls just because of the game; even though the players associated with that game are friends and sit back, watch and laugh at the fans getting into fights.

It doesn't matter what part of the country or countries that you live in, sports plays a major part in the economy. The local community hosting the big events always gets a major boost from that weekend due to the amount of tourism. The restaurants in that local area all see a spike as well as local shops. Flipside of that coin though is the amount of people that have to be hired for security and extra security that's needed for the events.

By events I'm not talking just about the Super Bowl, World Series, or championship games; I'm also talking about NASCAR events. I'm also talking about your local amateur events even though they may be smaller in scale. At one time NASCAR was able to keep up with other sports but the fan base of actually going to the races is in a decline due to the cost of the events and the cost of hotel rooms tripling; plus factor in that now you can't go to just one race, you pretty much have to do all the races. If you get rain during the weekend and they postpone the race, now you have to miss work one day and most just can't afford to take that chance.

We won't discuss fantasy sports that much, but that's a big thing nowadays. Be active and play the sports, but do it with caution.

Stimulants

Even though we've already covered some of the stimulants that are highly addictive, we still have to touch base on what exactly a stimulant is. A stimulant is an upper that causes a temporary amount of high alertness and energy. Most of the drugs that you find on the street including cocaine and Ritalin are stimulants.

When coming down off the high, the user will find themselves groggy, filled with depression and apathy. New addicts will quickly try to fill that void by using the stimulant again due to it being a short term usage. Over the course of time though, once the addiction takes over, users will experience an irregular heartbeat and a sense of hostility and extreme cases of paranoia.

As mentioned with many of the other drugs covered in the book, addiction is a serious issue because of the activity. You get used to wanting to chase that high without wanting to experience the low. Once we can get ourselves away from chasing that high to begin with, and settle with what we have going, everything will work out and we will no longer be chasing that high that the drugs give us. We don't need to hit that high level to experience the downfall.

Various

We're almost done with the types of addictions that we're going to cover in this book and then we'll get into teaching how to win the battle against addiction. There's a whole list of types of addiction that we didn't really get to cover and there's at least a thousand more; we're not covering every single one of them. We'll just cover a couple that are starting to hit the market now more than ever.

One of the first types of addiction that we're going to face here is what's known as bath salts. Bath salts are signed as an illegal drug thanks to the Obama administration but the use of the drug is on the rise. It has a longer stay in the system and can take up to 8 hours before coming down off the high. Some of the effects include fast heart rate, seizures, cold sweats and extreme paranoia to name a few. It usually comes in a bag of 500mg with a warning of "not to be consumed by humans" but that hasn't stopped people from experimenting. The usage of the drug doesn't show up on drug tests, but the amount of deaths due to overdose is on the rise.

Another drug that is on the rise is known as flakka and turns the user into a zombie like phase as well as organ shutdown. It's new to the market.

One of the newest drugs to hit the US in the past recent years is something known as krokodile. I didn't misspell it, that's how it is. This drug is extremely dangerous because within a couple short usages, your body is already on shutdown mode. Your skin can become infected with gangrene as well as skin ulcers. For those who have never heard of this drug, it's basically codeine, gasoline, and paint thinner and another item that's all mixed together and then injected.

Next up will be in the infamous love drugs; Ecstasy, Molly, and LSD. These drugs are illegal but college kids still find a way to get their hands on them for parties and they are still found at Raves. The problem is that not only are these lethal when combined, they create a false sense of reality and can lead to serious consequences. Ecstasy isn't around too much anymore but that's because they change the compound every couple years and bring it out with a new name. LSD has been around for the longest of times and will forever be involved. It's an acid and can be a tablet or on a strip. Crush any of these up at a college party and now you have a roofie, or even worse comes an incident that involves date rape.

There's more but already touched base on some.

Video Games

In today's society, the world of video games have taken over everyone from ages 10 all the way up to early to mid-60. We no longer in the day where it's about board games with the family or going out until the street lights come on. Video games are everywhere from cell phones, tablets, computers and video game systems. They consume life and have turned kids into walking games and have led to death.

Consider the most recent game that came out called Pokemon Go. This game has caused people to walk out in traffic blindly and caused riots for people to try to catch characters.

Video games aren't just about the exercise though that they can help provide. They've also created horrible outcomes with huge amounts of crime. There's something about playing a free roaming video game that involves killing random people and stealing cars, and selling drugs. Factor in a kid who's not happy with the situation that he's in and then goes out and recreates the game. It has happened not just in the US, but throughout the world. History has shown us that there are some people who think games can provide a life on the outside. Life isn't a video game, nor should it be treated like one.

On the flipside of that coin though, there are some games that can provide a real life experience. There are simulation games and sports games that real athletes and people in professional fields that help them hone their craft. We too as fans and fellow gamers get the chance to play the same game for prizes and other experiences. With simulators such as the NASCAR, NASA or the Flight Simulators, some fields *require* you to take your training through advancement on them before you can even step foot in the real world job. It's not just one time and in either; you are doing multiples and multiples of it before you're even thought of. To obtain a driver's license, you have to do a simulator *and* go through testing. Most of the Drivers Education courses now have simulators before they take you on the road.

While the argument can be made that video games can be good or bad, they still consume our life. Kids are now considered anti-social now because they'd rather play a multi-player video game at all hours of the night instead of homework or hanging out with friends. The video games re-launch the same game with different years slapped on the cover forcing you to buy the same game over and over. It's a monopoly and they have us hook line and sinker.

This will conclude our chapter on things that we can or have been addicted to. As you could tell already, most of the book dealt with some addictions that were harder than others, and not done by example. The book is done to show that no matter what we go through in life, we all suffer from one addiction or another. We are all going through the same issues, just deal with them differently.

I know it was a lot to take in and hopefully you're still with me as we now prepare to get over the addiction and start to get on the road to a better and healthier life. The remainder of the book will show you how to get through this lovely thing that we call life and will help you be able to manage it and get away from the part that we call **Rock Bottom**.

It will be a difficult challenge, but with the right amount of time and effort whether it be on your part or the person that you know that has the addiction, life can get better. The next chapter will be a way that will help you when dealing with withdrawals and will start with the recovery process. That's exactly what the rest of this book will be, a way to help the recovery start to take form. Following the rest of the book will guide you to doing what needs to be done. Again, I'm not in the field, I, too was an addict and found these to help me.

Chapter 3: Resist the Craving

There are a few things that we can do to get past the withdrawals that will make our lives a bit less difficult. When it comes to going through withdrawals, it's our mind sending signals to our body because it's craving that high. If we can get in the mind on our own, we don't need to medicate the problem. The thing is with that, our mind is and can be a very dangerous place to visit. Those who have never taken drugs are said to even only use a slight percentage of the brain.

But when we look at all of us having dealt with an addiction at one point of our life or another, it becomes a question of; how did or how can we beat that addiction? Some addictions are easier to beat then others; the length of time that you're hooked on the addiction can and will make a difference on how easy it'll make it. Your age will also play a factor in battling the cravings.

The argument can be made at times about what really is **Rock Bottom**. Rock bottom doesn't have to really be when you're at your lowest point in life, but can be described as when you feel all hope is lost. It can be a time when you feel guilt or remorse. It can be when you're in financial troubles. Let's get into the ways to get out of the withdrawals and start recovery.

The first way to deal with withdrawals is more of an analogy but has proven to work. In the very first book that I wrote called **Free the Mind**; I referenced to something that allowed us to release our inner thought process without having to overthink issues. Instead of saying to go on Amazon and buy the book, I'm going to put that analogy here.

Imagine your life being a movie. Everyone you know from the past and present is in that same theater with you sharing your moments whether they are happy, sad, and blank or fulfilled, courageous or embarrassing. Part way through the movie comes on about the addiction and that fills the remainder of the film. The lights come up and give you a chance to talk to everyone in the theater. You give a prolonged speech about making a change; a sacrifice of sorts. There are things in life that will be cut out and it may affect some people more than it will others. There are two doors to go out of the theater. One which will be the usual routine that happens day in and day out; and the other door is the one of change. The door of a new beginning with no looking back; which is the door you **must** exit through first. The relief that will follow will be a feeling that will be one like no other. You'll find some trying to stop you; just keep going on your path.

To continue with this analogy briefly, you have the power to decide for yourself as an addict or someone who's familiar with an addict to choose what it is that you're trying to accomplish. We can make that decision here and now to walk away from the bad and start fresh with something new. Everything in our past will still try to tempt us, but with our own personal strength and the power of the mind, we can get away from whatever addiction ails us. After we make the decision to go with a new beginning, our families will follow and find a stronger bond. We may lose some friends; even ones that we've known for years but that's the chances that we have to take. It's not the loss of the friendships; it's that we are changing our surroundings and what it is that we're doing, not just internally but externally.

Cravings can last an average time length of 20 seconds up to 4 minutes; pending on what the addiction was that caused the craving. When we feel that craving come on, it's important that we think of a happy place **prior** to what it was that caused the addiction. We can do yoga or meditation, go for a drive, talk to someone or find a hobby as well. The power of thoughts though can most definitely get us away from that craving, especially if it's a pain.

Somebody who deals with a pain medication addiction will have a harder time getting over the cravings than say someone who has a shopping addiction or a caffeine addiction. That's led to the fact that when someone has a pain, they automatically reach for something whether it's OTC or prescribed regardless of the size of the pain. It's not so much that it's their fault, it's because that's what they were trained to do from the time they can remember.

Dealing with pain, they can't just turn down a different road. When one pain dissipates, another one forms. There are a couple different things that we can do to rid the aches and pains. First and foremost as I mentioned in that part of the chapter, there are simple natural remedies that we can that are better for us. If we don't want to take natural remedies, we can look to doing meditation which allows us to tap into the pain through our minds and put the pain at ease.

In case you haven't noticed yet, when dealing with cravings, we can resist the temptation by using our inner minds. We don't need to go to the doctors and be prescribed medication. We don't need to pay a clinic. We need to figure out what we need to do for ourselves versus what we want. Even by going to the doctors it's a temporary relief. We don't *need* that.

When it comes to dealing with life and what we want to expect out of it, we can replay back to the shopping addictions. Life really is a precious thing and when dealing with the cravings and addictions in general, the key battle in this is the struggle of wants versus needs as I just recently mentioned.

We can be given anything we want to get that quick relief. Go to the clinics or doctors and they'll help us, yes but it's for a short time. When we come back out, roughly 72% have a rate to go back to doing what they went in for. It's not so much about being a repeat offender, and it's not that the person didn't want the change.

It's that the person who was suffering with addiction didn't notice the need for the change. They didn't fully notice the families that they have left behind to fulfill the craving and desire. When we can recognize what we want out of life and what we need to defeat the addiction, life will get 90% better. The last 10% will return in time and tempt us but with getting over the addiction, we can use the power to say no. It might even help the next person to get away from addictions, which we'll talk about later in the book. Addiction *is* a disease and we're all living with it. After the craving comes the motion of recovery.

Chapter 4: Stay Positive, Reject Negativity

After we resist the cravings and can get past the withdrawals starts the battle that we can dread as being an addict. Now we get the opportunity to face society head on with the fact that we are labeled as an addict. We have a few different options here and how we proceed will determine whether we stay strong or end up failing and going back to either being in the system or ending up dead at the worst case scenario.

One of the options that we have when dealing with society is to remind people that it's not who we are anymore. You'll still run into people who will say that "addicts are bad people" but they don't know that they too are suffering from the disease of addiction. They can argue with you left and right and say that we have a warped mind, but as you may have already read that **everyone** has an addiction at some point. We can tell people that we've turned a new leaf and they can either join in on who we are as a new person or they can sit back and watch. It's very important to remember that some of these people are the same ones who watched you fail and wouldn't do anything to help. These are the same people who want you to fail. Use that as a motivation! We are now in a positive state of mind and will continue to flourish.

We no longer have to deal with people who think negative of us. We know that while staying positive and thinking happy thoughts, we will no longer deal with negativity.

We'll still have a new kind of negativity to deal with; one that we haven't had to deal with yet and that's the stress level but stress is a lot easier to manage than the thought of going back to the addiction. We can't ever allow ourselves no matter how hard things may be to go back to the addiction that sent us down that hard path. If we do, it's not just the fact of facing the thought of being a failure, but also because the problems that we ran from will still be there. To handle the stress, remove yourself from the situation and close your eyes and do some controlled breathing. When you feel comfortable enough, then go back and face the issue in a controlled manner. If someone upsets you at the place of employment, take a quick break or just say you're running to the bathroom. This allows us time to breathe and a quick second away from whatever it is that's setting us off. If it's during a social activity, same thing; remove yourself and be the bigger person. There's no shame in walking away. There's no shame in dealing with what society is offering you to try to break you. It's kind of like a path.

One last analogy and then we'll get into the next step in our recovery process. This might help as it's helped others. Again, I'm not talking about just drug and alcohol addictions, its other types as well.

We as humans have the ability to dream and make our mind reach a brighter side to every outcome regardless of the situation. I'm sure you've heard the slogan "fork in the road," so let's take that and add something to it.

Put yourself in a dark secluded forest. You came in that forest through one path. Suddenly you reach a point where a thick stream of fog rolls in and you see that there's a fork and it can branch off into two separate paths. You're really not sure which one to take because you don't want to be lost, but you know that eventually you will find a way out. One path looks new and you can see a faint dimmer of light at the end of it even though it's covered in light fog. The other path doesn't have as much fog, but you can't see any light. Which path will you take? After going on the path with light fog, the light gets brighter and starts to show a glimmering promise of hope and comfort. You continue and find that it's the right path. Had you taken the other path, it would've led back to broken dreams. That's the power of positivity. Welcome to it.

Chapter 5: Winning the Battle

When we start to implement the things we are learning and can get over the new-found stress that will come into our lives; we can start focusing on the battle. This will be a battle that we can and will win from within. There will be no greater feat then when we can acknowledge that we did this on our own.

We've all heard the folklores of David and Goliath, Jack and the Beanstalk, and Oliver Twist to name a few. We've seen it in Hollywood films such as Rudy, Field of Dreams, the Express, and the Blind Side to name a few. We've seen it in real life where the underdogs always find a way to win, whether it's a team sport or it's an individual.

Just like the above mentioned, we are living an underdog story as an addict or someone who's in recovery. We are in the process of writing our own underdog tale as we are battling back from the addiction that knocked us out; so to speak. People can say that it's not the same to compare our lives to movies or to professional athletes, but aren't we overcoming the odds and beating the inner disease that's plagued us? Aren't we underdogs when trying to fight something that nobody else can see until it's too late; something that's "stronger" than what we are?

If we go into the rest of our life thinking that we're in the underdog role, there is nothing too steep that we can't defeat. We can worry about assembling a team later and surrounding ourselves with excellent people that will help us, but for now we really have to focus on ourselves. When we're done with ourselves, the rest will fall into place. We're not looking at just settling, we're looking at going above and beyond.

Before we go above and beyond though, we still have to do our routine and maintain the stay away from the addiction. Once we feel comfortable enough with ourselves, then we don't have to worry about anything else. Besides, if we can't be proud of ourselves, how can we expect others to notice what we're doing differently?

Winning the battle against addiction will get easier over time; that's a guarantee. If we do the right thing and continue to prove ourselves to the most important person (us) then we will get through it and then be able to focus on everything else.

Remember, addiction is a disease. Addiction is Goliath and with our hard work, our mental fighting of the disease, using some of the analogies, that we; *we* can tell our own personal tales of being David and slaying the giant and win the battle against addiction.

Chapter 6: Maintain the Fight

One of the greatest things about getting over addiction on our own is the ability to say "I told you so" and not be arrogant. You can be cocky that you beat the addiction, but don't want to get overzealous. There will still be temptations, pains, and other things that will come along that will make us want to relapse and get back into the disease. We just have to remember everything that we put into it and as the title of this chapter says; Maintain the Fight.

It doesn't matter how much time you have invested in your battle. It can be anywhere from one day to twenty years, we are all in the same boat. We can all face the same river that will force us to have to start downstream again and fight to get back up. Once we're able to overcome the struggles, we can become prone with certain things to say "it's only once, nobody will know" but that's not true; that's the furthest from the truth. We will know when we give up and go back to the ways that we used to be. We will know that we failed. We can tell others that we're doing great, but will lying get us anywhere; especially when we get caught? Is it really worth going back to the addiction to lose all the respect that we had just gained back from our peers and loved ones?

One of the things that we almost have to remember especially now is that we're not used to the "normal life." I say normal life because we got so used to resorting everything to our addiction as a healing. It's not like that anymore. Now it's about doing the right thing, keeping on the right path and maintaining everything that we fought for.

What really is normal to us now? Do we be content with where we are and what we do...or do we decide to take the chance and let ourselves go from being content? Can we recognize the differences that are happening; and when we do, can we make that jump? It's okay to want the new normal and live the normal life, but wouldn't it be better to live an abnormal life? A life of taking chances and experiencing new things at every possible chance? Life should be about spontaneous fun, not living in a routine. We don't have to worry about our friends and family finding out that we snuck back to our addiction because we beat the addiction. What we can do now is focus on helping someone else get over their addiction. We've already proven that everyone has an addiction to one thing at the minimum. We can now use the tools to help us maintain our personal fight by helping others fight their battles.

Chapter 7: Helping Others Win

What can be described as one of the greatest gifts that we have is the ability to help others. It doesn't matter if it's just with addiction, it's the fact that we are gifted with the presence of knowing when others are in trouble and seeing if there's anything we can do.

We can use this talent with addiction and other life skills. For the sake of conversation, right now we'll focus on addiction and get into the other life skills in a minute. When it comes to dealing with addiction and using **everything** that we've talked about in this book, it is very easy to notice when someone has an addiction. As we've been saying all throughout the book, addiction is a disease and it doesn't have to be just aimed at the usual suspects. We didn't even actually scratch the surface when it comes to types of addiction; this was just a brief topic of them. My point is a simple one; after getting our minds straight and seeing addiction for what it's worth, we can very easily see and want to help others with their own battle.

We can find different ways to be able to help them through their tough times when battling this disease. Different venues and times can play a factor. Not just help them, but it'll also help us.

When helping them get through their addiction, we have to be careful not to fall into the trap that can be laid to get us back into the spiral. Life can sometimes be a routine of ups and downs and as we learned and will continue to learn, it becomes easier to not get set up; but it's also easier to lax ourselves and get right back in the same ship.

When helping others get through the disease, we have to remember one simple rule; we are our first priority. We've already talked about the wants versus the needs and we can't force them to do something that they don't want to do; all we can do is show them the way and hope they'll join. Most of the times, people will want what we have and eventually will ask how to get it.

When people are at their **Rock Bottom** is when they are most open to seeing what life has to offer due to them being at the breaking point. It's also at the darkest point to where they see everyone going about their times and wonder why it's not happening to them. That's when we step in and try to offer encouragement and show them what we know. We don't need to be a counselor or a medical doctor to give them what they need to hear. It's not only a spiritual uplifting; it's a sense of pride for all involved.

Connecting to that is not just the field of addiction. When we are being positive that we succeeded in ourselves, the positivity will follow. We will see everything brighter, longer and stronger. Those who are around us will want to win with us. Regardless of the situation, it will work.

It doesn't matter if you're a rookie on a sports team or a seasoned vet, you can offer the sense of helping your fellow peers not just through encouragement, but also let's say they do something wrong. We can use our tools to casually walk up to them and talk to them about it that might help them get better at something. That will not only bring up their sense of morale and self-worth, but it'll make us feel good. They'll want to do the same and together we can be stronger.

If it's in the work force, you can help the next person coming along to get better. If it's somebody that's been there longer than you have, same thing; give them a helping hand. They'll return the favor and it'll make everything seem a lot easier and the days will pass quicker. It doesn't matter what kind of job that you're doing, it will get done faster and definitely will be a bit more pleasant. Take it from someone who works in retail at a grocery store; I see this all the time.

When you see a veteran or an elderly person, hold the door open for them; if it's a veteran shake their hand and thank them for their service. This is something that our younger generation has lost and don't see that much happening anymore. If you have the spare money and see a vet in line at your local coffee shop, buy them a cup of coffee or donut/bagel. They'll pass the favor onto someone else in time. Even if they don't, you have to remember that by helping others, we get that general sense of joy in our life because after we're going; they're still thinking about us. That one minute interaction in life can and will make someone's day a lot easier.

If you're at the line at a grocery store and see someone with only one item, offer to let them go in front of you or better yet; if it's inexpensive like a loaf of bread, pay for it. If you remember a couple years ago, one of the biggest movements was known as "Pay It Forward." This is sort of like what I'm talking about. The movement can be brought back, but see; when we're doing this and helping others, you never know who it is that you could be saving. The most important person that you're saving by doing this; is yourself. I promise you that you will not find any other greater joy in life other than using your cure to help others.

While we're wrapping up the book, and before I do my shout-outs to people who helped me get to where I'm at; I want to do a couple of follow ups and reminders and key points.

First and foremost, life is a precious gift and I know that it sounds like a preaching so to speak. It can be and probably is. However, in the same sense, it's really not. We have the tools and skills in our lives that we can use to overcome any obstacle that's thrown in our direction. We just have to use them to the best of our ability. We can walk the Earth alone and be bored, but if we use the power of our mind, we will never be bored. We will never visit the same place twice and never be in the same boring routine. It's about what we make of it and what we choose to do.

We have to battle addiction through ourselves and provide the strength to get through every day without having to resort to the last means. Whatever it is that ails us, we can and will overcome it. Some addictions are okay to have, but when we still use the sense that addiction is a disease, we'll find different ways to want to go through life without the disease. We don't have a warped mind; we weren't born with one so we don't have to use one to get through this journey known as life.

Every aspect of life and how it's presented to us is a great thing. All we have to do really is be wary of our surroundings and continue to do what's best for us and the rest of the things that's going to happen will. We can't get through life by having to resort to the addiction and live a healthy meaningful life. We have to be prosperous and let society see us for who we *are*, not what we were.

We can get out of the bottomless pit that's known as **Rock Bottom** by following the simple steps:

Recognize and Admit the Problem
Resist the Cravings
Work the Mind
Stay Positive and Reject Negativity
Win the Battle
Maintain the Fight
Help Others Win Their Battle

That's going to conclude the book. I really hope this helped you or someone you know be able to battle addiction. Again, I'm not in the medical field and everything that's listed here is what I've learned and done in my personal life to get away from my addictions. Thanks for reading and feel free to reach me if you have any questions or concerns.

Chapter 8: Closing and Shout-outs

Helena S. – There are so many words I wish that I can say to you but the most important words are; thank You. In the amount of time that we've known each other, and the ups and downs, you are a true inspiration. I can't even describe how you've helped me and so many others. You are truly a one-of a kind special girl and I look forward to many more memories with you. I can't wait for the next chapter.

Family – Thank you for your undying support and allowing me to become who I am. Through thick and thin, the journey of life continues and the level of knowledge continues. Thank you for letting me continue to follow my passions and being there with me and not giving up. Much love to each of you.

Jeri Rich and Mel – The memories that we share will forever be a part of me. I often tell everyone that you all are my second family, and in actuality it's how I see you. Between the advice, the fellowship and bonding that we all share, the life and times that have been shared will continue to grow. Love you guys and can't wait for the next chapter in our lives.

Donnie, Betsy and Jimmy – Words can't even begin to describe how much you guys mean to me. The fun that we have during Wednesday night bowling league and then the after-party gives a whole new meaning to excitement. Between the inside jokes and the amazing amounts of laughter, thanks for making bowling great again.

Chad, Mark, Willis, Dan, Gabe, Phil, Sheila, Doug, Jackie, Rob, and the rest of Gals and Guys league – Thank you for the support and the amazing fun times that we all get to share. It's always great to have at least one night a week to look forward to. The friendships and the amazing support that everyone has for each other is one that can't be mirrored that I've ever seen.

Sponsors – Thank You from the bottom of my heart for giving me the opportunity to continue to follow my dreams and not giving up. Not just in the sports aspect of life, but with staying with me through thick and thin and allowing me to stay with the path that I've chosen. I continue to hope to make you proud of what I'm doing and together this journey will continue to provide great travels. The best is yet to come.

Extended Friends and Family – Some of you whom I've talked to wanted to remain anonymous and I kept my promise. This book has changed a lot of our lives as it was being made and you have no idea how much you mean to me with the amount of support you've given. There were some times that it was beginning to be a struggle just because of the topic, but you kept my head in the game and made me see it though and for that I will forever be grateful. With not just going by the formation and the stuff that's in the book, but some of the life lessons that you've shown me will continue to stay with me for the remainder of my life. The skills that have been given will someday hopefully help someone else with their battles. Thank you for your continued support and we're moving on to the next one.

All things are possible when you have faith and continue to live your life through the Almighty God. When strength is needed, don't be afraid to ask for assistance; when there is victory, don't be afraid to give praise; when there is darkness, don't be afraid to ask for the light.

That concludes the book and I hope it helps you or helps someone you know find the better way.

www.ingramcontent.com/pod-product-compliance
Lightning Source LLC
Chambersburg PA
CBHW062342280526
45787CB00012B/584